I0478407

Webcam Savvy
For
Telemedicine

By
Clarence Jones

FIRST EDITION

Copyright © 2017

Webcam Savvy
For
Telemedicine

by Clarence Jones

First Edition
(also available as an e-book)
ISBN-13: 978-1546501893
ISBN-10: 1546501894

Other books by Clarence Jones

Winning with the News Media -
> *A Self-Defense Manual When You're the News*

They're Gonna Murder You -
> *War Stories from My Life at the News Front*

Webcam Savvy -
> *For the Job or the News*

Filming Family History -
> *Saving Great Stories for Future Generations*

Sailboat Projects -
> *Clever Ideas and How to Make Them*

More Sailboat Projects
> *Clever Ideas and How to Make Them*

Webcam Savvy for Telemedicine

Table of Contents

What is Telemedicine, Anyhow?

This shot is taken from a real Skype® interview aired by a TV network several years ago. In color, it's even worse than it appears here. In color, everything is tinged blue or pink.

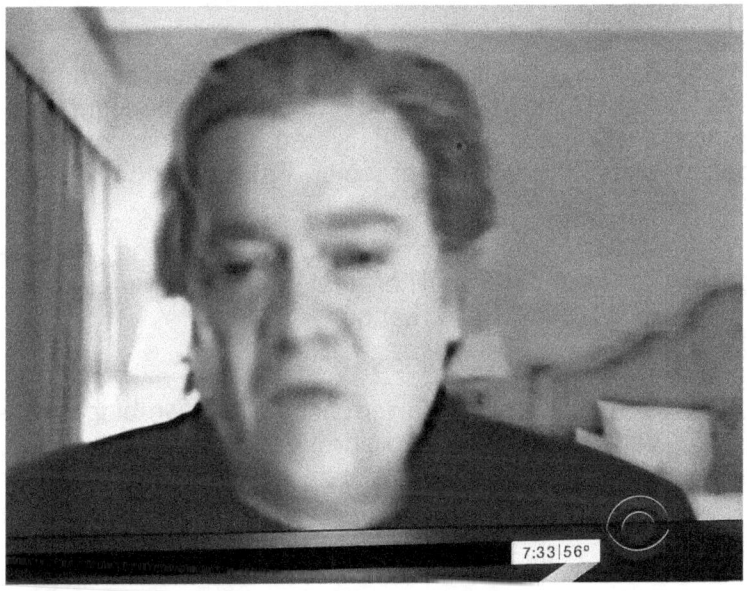

Nothing in the video is in focus. The network logo, the time, and temperature in the lower right are sharp, but they were superimposed over the image.

It appears to have been shot with a laptop webcam in a motel room. Awful. Truly awful.

So bad, viewers probably didn't hear a word this guy spoke. The Gettysburg address would have been overwhelmed by the miserable setup.

Times Have Changed

It is this kind of setup that makes doctors, nurses and patients shy away from Telemedicine. But times have changed. Today's equipment is astounding. It will soon revolutionize medicine. I'll show you what it can do. And how to use it.

A Simple Definition

The simplest definition of Telemedicine is:

> The transmission of medical information from one place or person to another – especially the examination of a patient by a doctor or nurse, connected through the Internet, in real time.

There are unspoken nuances in the Telemedicine term.

It is more than just the DELIVERY of medical information. Medical information has been delivered for centuries. Usually by mail. Sometimes hand-delivered. By courier, or by the patient. From the lab to the doctor. From one doctor to another.

Telemedicine is much more. It involves technology – a machine, a system or a pipeline – that can transmit medical information in a two-way exchange.

Telemedicine's Advantages

- Convenience and lower cost are the two biggest advantages for Telemedicine.
- You can connect at any time, just about any place in the world. Distance is no longer a factor.
- There is no need for an appointment, no need for transportation, no delay in diagnosis and treatment.
- Once they're comfortable with it, patients tend to check in more frequently and ask more questions.
- Doctors and nurses can do a better job of follow-up care with Telemedicine.
- Telemedicine can sharply reduce the cost and patient overload in hospital emergency rooms.

Emergency Room Overloads

About half the people who go to emergency rooms are not having an emergency. Most don't even need urgent medical attention. But federal law says the ER can't refuse to see and treat them. Even if they can't pay for a doctor to deal with their headache or indigestion.

Resistance to Telemedicine

Among doctors, there is a lot of resistance to the Telemedicine idea. Let's see if we can figure out why.

In the 1800s, surely telegraph wires must have transmitted some medical information. But if they did, it was rare.

In the early 1900s, newspapers developed ways to transmit photographs. First, by telephone lines, then with radio signals. But the technology was not good enough to transmit medical information with life and death significance.

Telephone Calls & Fax Machines

Then doctors began to talk to their patients - and to each other - by telephone. Was that Telemedicine? Yes.

Once they were perfected in the 1960s, fax machines were regularly used to send medical records. Telemedicine? Yes.

We have reached the point now where X-rays are routinely sent to radiologists halfway around the world to detect and diagnose terminal diseases. The quality of the X-ray at the receiving end is identical to the quality of the original.

Medical Care for Remote Areas

The largest single benefit provided by Telemedicine worldwide is medical attention for those in remote areas who simply cannot get to a doctor or medical clinic.

This is the case in many developing, sparsely populated countries with very few doctors and medical facilities. Some are island nations. In others, the terrain is so mountainous, travel to a doctor or medical facility can take many days.

Telemedicine now offers consultation with specialists for rural areas in the United States, where there are only family doctors practicing general medicine. Most Americans are unaware of Telemedicine because they have such easy access to highly sophisticated, in-person medical care.

Why Doctors are Reluctant

Despite all that, there is still a great deal of reluctance among American doctors to use Telemedicine for the diagnosis and treatment of patients.

Why are doctors so reluctant?

- Because this is new. Any major change in medicine is extremely difficult to accomplish. It takes a while.
- Doctors are not sure they will be paid. Medicare, Medicaid and other insurance systems are beginning to work out ways to guarantee payment.
- Doctors are afraid their diagnosis by telemetry will miss something they would catch if they examined the patient in person. They could be sued for malpractice, or lose their license.
- Most have not seen the astounding quality of audio and video that Telemedicine now offers.
- Some state laws do not recognize Telemedicine, and doctors there are waiting for the law to change.

There are so many companies moving into Telemedicine, clever solutions to deal with these problems are multiplying.

This Book Can't Keep Up

The move to Telemedicine is so massive, any attempt in this book to explore the latest developments would be out of date before the ink dries. Market researchers predict the Telemedicine industry will reach about $2 billion in 2018, and grow another $1 billion per year after that.

So this book provides:

- *Telemedicine Resources* - a chapter to help you find on the Internet what happened yesterday in Telemedicine or became the norm today.

- *Telemedicine Tools* - another chapter that will show you some of the clever tools now available for examining patients online.

- How to develop the personal, on-camera skills for doctors, nurses and patients that are necessary for successful Telemedicine.

- How to purchase and set up inexpensive equipment at both ends so both patient and care providers can practice, and hone their webcam skills.

Practice, Practice, Practice

Please excuse the old saw:

> TOURIST in New York asks a stranger on the sidewalk, "How to you get to Carnegie Hall?"

> ANSWER: "Practice, practice, practice."

Communicating effectively on camera (instead of in-person) also takes a lot of practice. Because something happens subconsciously when you're on camera.

When I moved from newspapers to television, an old friend who worked in TV took me aside for some helpful advice:

> "When I see you on television," he said, "You look like you're making a speech to the Orange Bowl. That's because you're thinking of a million people out there in the audience."

Changing Your Mind-Set

The audience, he said, is only one or two people. They're sitting eight or 10 feet away from the TV set, in their family room or kitchen. So as you speak, you have to imagine them, sitting there, very close, in that tiny space, as you explain something to them.

Once I learned how to shift my mind-set, I became a much better communicator.

A patient's visit with a doctor or nurse requires the same kind of shift in mind-set. To be effective, both people have to imagine that the camera is the other person in a conversation that is taking place in a doctor's office, a hospital or a clinic.

More Difficult Than It Sounds

This is much more difficult than it sounds.

And it takes practice. Luckily, webcam technology has reached the point where extremely good equipment is affordable, easy to use, and perfect for that learning experience.

Most people who are computer-savvy have already tried Skype (freeware, provided by Microsoft®) or Face Time® (the Apple® equivalent).

With those programs, you can record sessions, then go back and replay them to hone your skills.

When I left reporting I became an on-camera coach, working with government and corporate executives all over America. I am convinced that watching video of your own performance is the most effective learning technique ever invented.

We Deceive Ourselves

I also learned that we are very good at self-deception. Looking at the replay, the person on camera often will not see quirks that others pick up immediately.

Very few of us are born with these on-camera skills. So it always helps to have a friend watch with you, as a candid, sometimes brutal critic.

The Right Equipment

For the practice sessions, you will need to use a good webcam, microphone, background and lights. You can set this up easily for less than $200. I'll show you how.

One reason Skype interviews have such a bad reputation is that they were shot with built-in webcams. Not good.

We have become so accustomed to slickly produced video on television, most Skype interviews scream AMATEUR-BEGINNNER. Because they're:

- Filmed with a low-quality webcam
- Shot at a strange angle
- Poorly framed
- Badly lit, with a cluttered background of
  - Debris and
  - The sound of a crying baby or a barking dog

The New Norm

Webcam interviews are rapidly becoming the norm for many business, news, and government agencies. They save a lot of staff time, travel, and money.

But in terms of quality, they're often lousy. They are today's equivalent of kids playing telephone with tin cans connected by a string.

That's why moving to Telemedicine can seem like such a difficult hurdle. Compared to the slick packaging of TV news, webcam results can be downright weird.

The Webcam Filter

Corporations realize the webcam process for job interviews has limitations. So they use it as a filter to eliminate those who obviously don't fit what they're looking for. Most companies still use face-to-face interviews for the finalists.

The Same Criterion for Medicine

The same protocol applies for doctors and nurses in Telemedicine. Triage in Telemedicine should decide which patients need to be seen in person. For those judgments you need the right equipment and know how to use it.

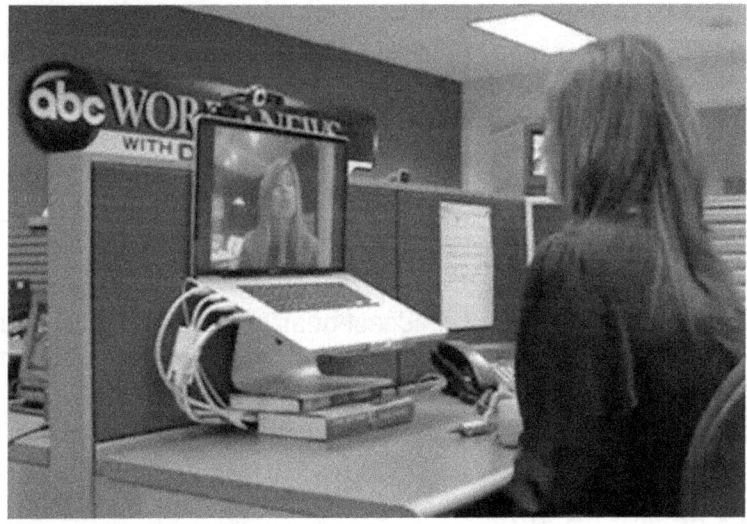

Solutions Often Very Simple

Telemedicine solutions can be very simple, compared to everyday medical procedures. Here's an example. This network correspondent has used two books to raise her laptop on the desk so the tiny camera built into the top rim of her laptop screen will be at her eye level. Crude, but it works.

TV News Only Needs Quality at One End

For the TV news interview by webcam, the shot of the reporter is not nearly as important as the video of the person being interviewed.

If we see the reporter at all in the edited story, she will probably re-shoot the video of her asking questions with a broadcast-quality camera in the newsroom. In TV news, that's called "shooting reverse questions."

Telemedicine Needs Quality at Both Ends

Telemedicine interviews must have quality at both ends of the conversation.

The doctor or nurse needs high-quality audio and video to do a good job of diagnosis and treatment.

The patient needs to see high quality at the other end to feel that the visit, diagnosis and treatment were as good as they would have been in person.

If a physician or medical facility decides to go into Telemedicine, the equipment will be supplied by a company that has built into it the necessary security that HIPAA requires.

Meanwhile, the patient, the doctor and the nurse can develop their camera skills with simpler, cheaper gear.

You Won't Like the Way You Look

If you've been interviewed in person by a TV news crew (reporter, photographer, broadcast-quality camera, lights and microphone) you probably didn't like the way you looked and sounded. Even with all those pros and expensive gear.

Just wait until you see and hear yourself for the first time on Skype or Face Time.

TV Interviews Unfair

TV news interviews in person have always been unfair. Stress can look like guilt, or fear, or deception.

In a Telemedicine interview, the obvious discomfort of a doctor or nurse screams into the camera: I DON'T REALLY KNOW WHAT I'M DOING.

Exams by Medical Students

That's why learning through practice is so important. If you're a doctor or nurse, you probably remember your first patient exams when you were a student.

Most medical and nursing students are terribly uneasy.

And the patients are just as uncomfortable, knowing they're being examined by an amateur.

In Telemedicine, if you're a doctor or nurse, you need to exude confidence and professionalism. That takes practice.

If you're the patient, you need to learn how to talk to the camera so the doctor or nurse will pick up all the visual clues they need to provide the care you need.

This book is designed to help at both ends.

Rent a Webcam

Consulting companies are popping up that will help organizations that want better results with webcam interviews.

For a fee, the specialty service company overnights a high-quality webcam and microphone to the interviewee, with detailed instructions on how to set them up.

After the event, the equipment is shipped back to the consultants.

Even with the consulting company's fee, the cost can be much lower than travel for an in-person interview.

Working with top quality equipment, you're still at a disadvantage if you don't know how to use it. For many businesses and professions, webcam savvy is rapidly becoming a survival skill.

You probably already own a laptop with a built-in webcam. To get up to speed and practice for Telemedicine exams, you need to use another webcam (about $70) that will plug into a desktop, laptop or tablet.

Incredibly Easy to Use

Surprisingly, the latest webcams have improved so much, they approach broadcast quality. And even if you're intimidated by electronics, they are incredibly easy to use.

In the following chapters, I'll show you how to create winning Telemedicine interviews and exams.

What's Ahead for Doctors & Nurses

- On-camera skills that make patients like, believe, and trust you
- How these skills can make you the "doctor on call" when TV news needs a quick medical opinion. It's free advertising. And good for your practice. It can also build trust and confidence from your patients.
- Why a fast computer and Internet connection are crucial
- How to choose the right webcam
- How and where to buy it at the best price
- Installing and setting it up
- Lighting your set
- Creating a background to reinforce your message and not distract from it

What's Ahead for Patients

There are some patients whose conditions need constant oversight. Many of them simply cannot travel to a medical facility on a daily basis.

Telemedicine is a WONDERFUL solution for those cases.

A webcam can be set up in their home, where they feel comfortable. Even if they live alone and have never used a computer, they can easily learn how to use a webcam.

The doctor or nurse has the ability to tell the patient what's needed as the exam progresses.

If the patient has a caregiver at home, or lives in a nursing facility, that other person can be a superb assistant for a Telemedicine exam.

On Camera Skills for Doctors and Nurses

Nothing works better on camera than <u>sincerity</u>. Most people fall short because they don't know how to be sincere to a camera.

Following closely behind sincerity is <u>caring</u>. You MUST make it obvious that you care about the patient.

Convincing patients that you sincerely care about them is probably the most critical (and sometimes most difficult) Telemedicine skill to master.

Medicine has always called that "bedside manner." It cannot be automatically transferred to a camera. In this different setting, it must be learned all over again.

In the *Practice, Practice, Practice* chapter, I write about changing your mindset by imagining that the camera is your patient.

Making Love to the Camera

I remember watching the British actor Michael Caine being interviewed on *The Today Show*. The BBC was filming a series of documentaries called "Masters of Their Craft." Caine had been chosen as a master of the acting craft.

"How did you learn to be a master craftsman?" the interviewer asked.

"I learned how to make love to the camera," Caine responded.

"What do you mean?" he was asked.

"Watch," Caine said.

Suddenly He Changed

And suddenly he changed. He was still the same person, but different. He was warmer. The voice was more intimate. The eyes had a new twinkle.

He was someone you'd like to spend time with; exchange secrets with. He exuded sincerity.

In teaching on-camera skills I sometimes tell clients to imagine that the camera is the love of their life. You're on your first date. He or she is sitting across the table in a restaurant. Turn on your charm. You want that person to like you. Believe you. Trust you.

Loss of Energy

One of the hurdles here is the subtle loss of energy that occurs when we watch someone on camera. I have interviewed thousands of people on camera.

And almost without exception, when I watched the replay, they were not as lively, not as engaging, not as effective as they were, live, when I filmed the interview.

I know the camera is accurate. The camera has not distorted time or facial expression. It has not siphoned away sincerity or caring.

No. Something happens in the *perception of the viewer*.

The Face Formula

In the chapter ahead on *Creating Sound Bites*, you'll find my FACE formula. At the risk of being repetitive in that chapter, I'll tell you now that the E in that acronym stands for ENERGY.

You may have had the experience of time slowing down in moments of great stress. It can happen as your car goes into a skid. Or you face a robber with a gun.

Tachypsychia

The technical term for this is tachypsychia. It is caused by:

- A dump of adrenalin in your bloodstream
- Total, focused attention

It is my theory that people are more boring on camera than they are in real life because the viewer has to focus more on what is being said than they would if the conversation was taking place in person.

Focusing on the screen causes a slight bit of tachypsychia. So you must invest more energy on camera, to correct the distortion. How much energy?

The only way to know is to watch yourself on camera. And then practice until you know, as you speak, what you're projecting. As you invest more energy, you need to <u>appear</u> that you're speaking in your normal tone of voice.

Directing the Patient

In a Telemedicine exam, you will need to direct the patient, or someone with the patient, With most software, they have a small window on their screen that shows them what you're seeing. But they need directions. Like:

- "Can you move a little closer to the webcam so I can see that place on your cheek a little better?

- "Yes, hold your arm right there for a moment. I want to take a picture of it."

- "Can you walk across the room now, then turn and come back? I need to see how that broken ankle is doing."

Tools Patients Can Use Alone

In the upcoming chapter on *Telemedicine Tools*, I show equipment already available for long-distance exams that patients can use without assistance. You may need to say:

- "Now I want you to pick up that stethoscope and hold it against your chest so I can hear your heart."

- "Just a little to the left. Good. Now take in a deep breath and hold it." OR

- "You have a tool there that looks like a ballpoint pen with a wire on it. The other end has a little light. I'd like you to put the light inside your left nostril and hold it while I look around in there."

- "Now open your mouth wide, and point the light at the back of your throat as you say Aaaah."

"On the Side of God & the Angels"

I also believe in mantras to help you communicate better.

I tell clients who are preparing for court testimony to repeat over and over on the way to the courthouse:

"I am on the side of God and the angels. I am going to speak truth today to bring light and justice to the world."

For a difficult patient, you may need to get yourself ready before the Telemedicine session begins. Like thinking:

> *This is an elderly patient, with a great deal of arthritic pain. I am going to be the most charming, delightful doctor she has ever talked to. Nothing she says will ruffle me.*

Learning to Say It Quickly

I suggested earlier that you make love to the camera. On that first date with the love of our lives we talked for hours.

But medical exams on camera are very short. The attention span for a Telemedicine patient is even shorter than one in person. I sometimes say to a client, "You know too much."

I have a one-liner:

> **The ultimate on-camera skill is learning how to tell the history of the human race in one sentence, without taking breath.**

The Elevator Speech

This has also been called "the elevator speech." Tell me what I need to know in the time it takes the elevator to go from one floor to the next.

Remember, the attention span on camera is very brief. If the patient wants to know more, they'll ask a follow-up question. You'll be given more time to expand your thoughts.

What to Wear

Dress the same as you would at work. For doctors, that usually means a white coat. For nurses, it can be scrubs. Medical schools seem to have taught you to always wear a stethoscope around your neck. So we'll know you're qualified.

Subtle Behavior You Need to Study

In the on-camera exam, there are subtle things that can dramatically affect how you're perceived. And the only way you can know what they are - for you - is to practice with a webcam and study the replay.

The traits below are GOOD/BAD. The first is usually considered good by most patients. But if you overplay them, they can give a bad impression. There is often a very thin line between them.

It can be a very slight inflection in your voice, facial expression or body English. These can be more noticeable on camera than in person. Here are some of them:

Walking the Tightrope

Self-confident/Arrogant

Aggressive/Overpowering

Hard worker/Workaholic

Empathetic/Maudlin

Precise and well organized/Obsessive-compulsive

Sense of humor/Takes nothing I say seriously

Humble/Meek

Cool, calm/Distant, uncaring

Decisive/Control freak

Enthusiastic/Wild and unpredictable

Cautious/Wimpy and afraid to try new things

Creative/Unmanageable

Patients More Forthcoming

Patients are often intimidated when they're talking to a doctor or nurse in person. They forget to ask questions they planned to ask before the exam.

A Telemedicine exam can be less intimidating. It seems easier to ask embarrassing or off-the-wall questions online than it is in person.

This is really apparent in the comment sections of items posted online. Some people become so uninhibited in the anonymity of the web, comments are shut down.

Use Lots of Graphics

I learned as a TV reporter how to double the audience retention for numbers and statistics. Use graphics. If you show visually what you're talking about as you speak, the listener will remember twice as much.

You may be surprised at how much more your patient understands and absorbs when you reinforce what you say with graphics.

How a New Drug Works

If you're telling a patient how a new drug works, try to find a drawing or photo. Print it, and hold it in front of the webcam.

If you're telling a patient recovering from a heart attack how important exercise will be for recovery, use charts and graphs that show how exercise affects survival rates

Revisiting Time with You

For patients with short memories or attention spans, they can record and replay the time they spend with you.

Especially sections they didn't quite understand when you covered them.

Patients often won't admit they failed to grasp something you said. With Telemedicine, they can privately go back and replay it until they DO get it.

Be the Doctor On Call

The on-camera skill you develop in talking to your Telemedicine patients can open a lot of new doors for you and your practice.

Television news is constantly looking for experts who can analyze and offer more insight in their stories. The networks have experts under contract who do this regularly. Medical, economic, legal, military, scientific experts.

Is Your Number In Their Contact List?

I tell my media relations clients that one of their primary goals should be to have their names and numbers in the electronic versions of the old Rolodex® system for every reporter and editor in their community.

When I was reporting for WPLG-TV in Miami in the 1980s, there was a stock broker who specialized in airline stocks. He was also very good at giving quick, concise interviews.

If anything happened that was connected to airlines or air travel, you could call, drive to his office, and interview him immediately.

The "Super" Billboard

Miami was a big city for airline news - gateway to Latin America - headquarters for several airlines - the site of some major crashes. The broker frequently appeared in those stories as an expert/analyst.

Every time one of those interviews was broadcast, his name and brokerage firm appeared on the "super" across his chest. He was a pioneer. Great advertising.

Medical Expertise

All of the national networks have doctors who are used as experts to help explain major medical stories.

Local newscasts would LOVE to have their own, local doctor to serve in that same capacity. But few doctors have the skill, inclination or time. If you go into Telemedicine, all that changes.

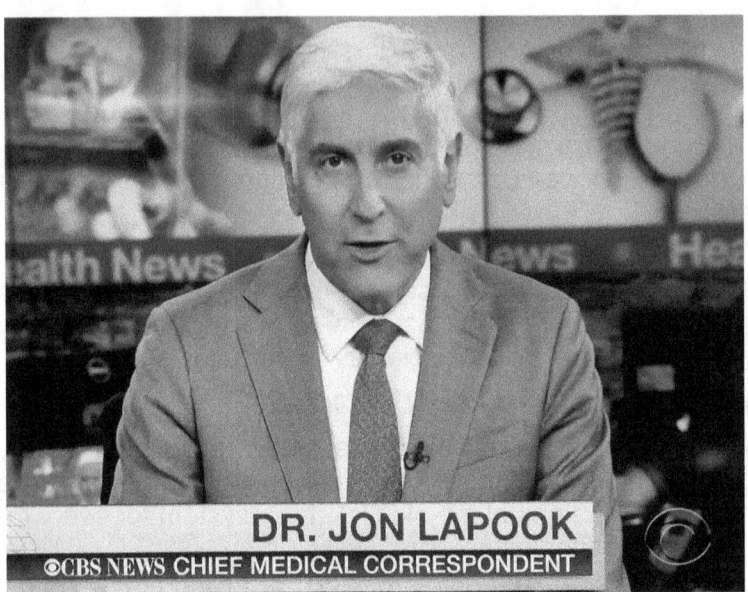

DR. JON LAPOOK
©CBS NEWS CHIEF MEDICAL CORRESPONDENT

Here is one of the network doctors on call, putting a new drug or procedure in perspective. The skills you develop for Telemedicine will make it easy for you to become the local doctor on call.

With the webcam in your office you can quickly connect to a reporter or anchor in a local TV station newsroom.

At a Time You Choose

Most of the time, the interview can take place any time you choose. It will be recorded for use on the evening news. The entire process will take less than 20 minutes away from your regular schedule.

Occasionally, they will want you to talk live with the anchors during the evening newscast. After your regular work day.

Being interviewed for a news story convinces your patients that you truly are an expert in your particular field. Otherwise, the TV reporter would not have included you in their story.

Some doctors and clinics buy commercial time on TV to advertise their specialties. When you're in a news story, the audience knows you didn't buy the TV time. A news interview makes you much more believable than a commercial would.

The Local News Peg

One of the most persistent, predictable kinds of news stories is a local story "pegged" to a national or international story. American editors are genetically programmed - absolutely compelled - to publish and broadcast these stories.

If America sends combat troops into a foreign country, local media MUST produce a story on whether or how local soldiers might be involved.

When a major bridge collapses, reporters all across the country write "pegged" stories about whether aging local bridges are safe.

When a breakthrough in cancer treatment is announced, the local TV audience wants to know whether that treatment is available locally, and where.

What is News?

One of the most succinct definitions of news:

> NEWS IS THE UNUSUAL.

If the headline says The Mayor Was Sober Today, it means that's unusual.

So reporters need experts who can tell us how unusual today's event really is. Their stories need a little history. An expert who knows the background, and predicts what it all means, is absolutely essential.

Credibility as an Expert

Experts interviewed for news stories are much more credible if their opinions will not affect them (or their competitors) financially.

This is why college professors are interviewed so often for news stories. Their education, knowledge and arm's-length experience are a given.

If we find out the expert on camera has a financial interest in the company that manufactures the product they're analyzing, believability can go down the tubes.

The Ethics of Expertise

So the expert should fully disclose up front anything that might even *suggest* a conflict of interest.

Medical school professors, for instance, should not provide their opinion or analysis of an experimental procedure in which they are involved. UNLESS they explain that at the top of the interview.

How to Become the Doctor on Call

If appearing in TV news stories as a medical expert appeals to you, here's how to do it:

- Read EVERY WORD in this book

- Buy and set up a high-quality webcam

- Create a "set" in your office where you can quickly be interviewed over the Internet

- When you see a story in which your opinion or analysis would be valuable, (especially if there is a local angle) call the news director of your favorite local TV station immediately

- They may not be aware of the local connection. Explain your expertise and what you could say if you were interviewed

- Tell him/her you have a high-quality webcam and could do the interview in the next 30 minutes

- If that news director is not interested, call another

- If the interview goes well, let the news director know you can be on call for future stories that involve your expertise

Don't Sell Too Hard

In that first contact, don't sell too hard. You'll make the news director suspicious. Suppose there is no breaking story the day you approach a local TV station. Call the news director and tell him/her you've developed on-camera Telemedicine skill, and have a webcam set up in your office.

Explain your education, experience and expertise, and your willingness to help them flesh out future stories in your field.

They'll probably want to audition you. If they don't seem interested, approach the news director at another station.

Delay Talking About Being Paid

It's usually best to not talk about being paid in your first conversations with a news director. That comes later. After they've used interviews with you several times, you'll have a working relationship with the news director.

They may make an offer before you bring it up.

If not, ask if other experts on call for the station are paid. If none are, you might shop around for another local station.

Suggest that you could be on call for quick interviews in your field with a title like "consultant" or "special correspondent." This kind of arrangement usually includes a written contract that pays you a set amount each time you appear.

Creating Your Set

Read the *Lighting and Background* chapter carefully. The chapter in this book- *Build a Backdrop Frame* - shows how to make a simple frame to hold a fabric backdrop. As an expert-on-call, you might want to work on something fancier.

If you teach at a medical school, practice at a hospital, or conduct research at a special laboratory, there will be a photographer whose portfolio includes pictures of the institution.

Or you can shoot it yourself. It's easy to have a wall-sized print made. Then hang it where it becomes the background when you're on camera.

The Pecking Order

You should understand how most local TV stations are organized. There is a GENERAL MANAGER (usually referred to by employees as the GM) who is responsible for everything at the station.

One of the department heads will be the NEWS DIRECTOR, who hires and fires reporters, editors and photographers. The news director sets general policy for news, but at large stations may not be personally involved in the gathering and production of most stories.

That's the job of the ASSIGNMENT EDITOR, who is usually the first person in the newsroom each day. The assignment editor reads the local newspaper to help create a list of the stories that will be in tonight's newscast.

The assignment editor decides which reporters and photographers will be assigned to produce each story.

Out in the Field

Out in the field, the photographer and sound technician work under the direction of the reporter.

As more advertising and news delivery moves to the Internet, many stations have had to drastically cut their newsroom budgets.

Digital video cameras are so much more automated than film cameras were, many local TV reporters are becoming a "one-man-band." If the union contract permits that.

The reporter works alone, and puts the camera on a tripod to shoot himself/herself for standups or reverse questions.

News Media Interviews

If you're a doctor or nurse, and Telemedicine interviews develop your on-camera presence, you may be in a position to become an advocate in the news media for your profession.

Those in medicine complain a lot about stuff like Medicare, Medicaid, insurance companies and too much paper work. But they are, IMHO, incredibly incompetent at organizing to change the things they dislike.

Like Herding Cats

"It's like herding cats," one of my doctors once said when I asked why he and other doctors were not better at working together to change the things that irk them.

I'm prejudiced, but I believe that organizing as advocates, and learning how to get your message across in the news media is the only way you'll ever bring about major changes.

Winning with the News Media

So I've included in this and the following chapter excerpts from the 9ᵗʰ Edition of my book, "*Winning with the News Media.*"

If this whets your appetite, the book is available in both print and Kindle formats at www.amazon.com .

All other e-book formats can be previewed and downloaded at www.smashwords.com .

If TV wants an interview, a reporter or producer will usually telephone to ask if you have a webcam. If you do, and they're in a hurry, they might want to call you back on Skype immediately to record the interview.

The first basic rule is:

RULE # 1 Give Yourself Time

Give yourself time to prepare.

If your pulse speeds up, pause. If the reporter's call makes your adrenaline surge and your breath quicken, you may be in Fight or Flight mode.

Under stress, you will not think well. Take some time to get your thoughts together. Make some notes. Most doctors and nurses have never been interviewed for a news story. It is a scary prospect. I'll try to make it less threatening.

What Does the Reporter Need?

The quotes that people regret are usually said reflexively, in the traumatic surge of surprise, anger or shock.

If you can stall for even 10 minutes, you'll do a better job of speaking for yourself and/or your profession.

Can I Call You Back?

So you say to the reporter or producer who's on the phone, "I'm really busy on something right now, but I think I can finish it in about 15 minutes. Can I call you back then?"

Which is true. You have some work to do to get ready for this interview. If that timetable works for them, get a quick grasp of what the story is about.

What do they want in this interview with you? Then hang up and spend the 15 minutes getting ready.

Everything in One Sentence

Use the time to decide what you really want to say. Boil it down to one sentence you can speak without taking a breath.

That one sentence will become the foundation of the interview. Other thoughts will branch out from it, but you'll want to keep coming back to it. Explaining it. Expanding it.

One of the great handicaps in doing a news interview is knowing too much about the subject. They don't have time for all you know. For this effort, you need to work on just that one, single thought.

Repeat the Central Idea

In normal conversation, if you repeat yourself, we wonder if you're getting senile. But in a news interview (that's being recorded, not live) if you say it often enough, at least one of those quotes or sound bites stating the central idea will almost certainly be used.

As a TV reporter, before a friendly interview, I would often say to my interviewee: "I may ask you the same question several times. It doesn't mean I'm not listening.

"That's a signal that I think you can give me a better, shorter answer. It means let's try that one again."

In normal conversation, we build up to our conclusion. We lay the groundwork first, before we get to the point. In media interviews, the process is reversed.

Always give the conclusion first. Then tell us how you got there. This takes practice. It is like telling a joke, punch line first.

Check With Staff

During that 15-minute reprieve before you make the webcam connection, check with your staff. "A reporter just called. The story they're pursuing caught me completely by surprise. Is there something I should know?"

The delay rule isn't necessary if the reporter's request is for simple information that poses no threat. But if you react viscerally, buy some time.

If the interview is critical to you or your organization, do it in person, if possible. Forget the webcam. It's much easier for you to get a handle on the reporter and the story angle if you're really face-to-face.

Personalities sometimes don't transmit accurately if the conversation is done electronically.

Make Sure It IS a Reporter

If you don't recognize the name or voice of the reporter on the phone and the story is sensitive, use the delay tactic. Before you hook up by webcam, make sure the call is legitimate.

The callback number the caller gave you may bypass the switchboard. So call the TV station or network's listed number and ask for the person who requested the interview.

Private detectives, insurance investigators, political operatives and business competitors sometimes pose as journalists. They'd love to catch you by surprise on video.

Ambushes by Webcam

If they know you always have Skype running in the background, you can be the victim of a webcam ambush - a surprise, instant video interview. If it's a TV reporter or producer, FCC regulations require them to tell you you're on the air.

Once you've agreed to be interviewed by webcam, and after you've done your homework, the next rule is:

RULE # 2 - The Pre-Interview-Interview

Conduct what I call a pre-interview-interview. From the first contact, where you arranged to delay the interview for a few minutes, you know generally what the story is about. When you call back, or when the webcam connection is made, expand that inquiry. Weave it into the social chat that begins most conversations.

Getting Acquainted

If you understand what the reporter is after, you can save a lot of time and anxiety. In this get-acquainted conversation, try to learn some basics:

- What exactly is the story assignment, and who thought it up?

- When will the story run, and what is the deadline for finishing it?

- How much time will the story be given?

- Who else has the reporter interviewed?

- Has any other research been done?

- How much knowledge does this reporter seem to have on this subject, and what kind of preconceptions?

- How intelligent and experienced does the reporter seem to be?

What is the Story About?

This is a very important thing you need to know, so you can judge whether the reporter is working on a preconceived, misguided concept. If that's the case, you'll have to work very hard to swing the story in another direction.

Particularly if the misconception came from the reporter's assignment editor or news director.

The reporter doesn't want to tell the boss the story idea was stupid. You'll have to work very hard to convince the reporter the boss' story concept should be abandoned.

Are They Here To Hurt You?

Before the real interview begins, you should have a good idea about whether the reporter will try to gut you, or simply needs your sound bites to fill out the story - to give it authority and credibility.

Young, inexperienced reporters are rarely given tough investigative assignments. If not done right, those stories can bring lawsuits. If the reporter seems very sharp, and seems to know a lot about the subject, that can be a warning flag.

As an investigative reporter, the interview with my target was my last stop before I wrote the script. I wanted to know as much as possible before the interview, so I'd know which questions to ask, and whether my target was lying.

The Play Dumb Con

Good investigative reporters can also con you into believing they're dumb and innocent, so you'll talk more freely. They'll respond with "no kidding?" or "really!" to things they already know. That makes you want to tell them more.

You may learn in the pre-interview interview that you need to gather some more written information to help you recall exact facts and figures.

A Great Opportunity

If you discover the reporter knows very little about the subject matter, you have a great opportunity to steer the story your way.

The way you structure the pre-interview conversation can strongly influence the questions when the real interview begins.

The interview may simply repeat the earlier conversation. That's all the new, inexperienced reporter knows to ask.

If the Reporter Offers, Take It

Many new reporters, uncomfortable with their lack of knowledge and skill, may even tell you in advance exactly what they're going to ask. If they make the offer, take it.

Remember: EVERYTHING is recorded. Avoid any asides that could easily become the story or change the way it's written. Anything you do or say can come back to haunt you.

Why Was That In the Story?

Avoid the temptation to educate the reporter too much. An inexperienced reporter may not be able to pick out the most important things you said.

"Why was that in the story?" you'll think when it's broadcast. Because you gave the information to the reporter. So stick to the topic and don't wander around. This gives you much more control of what's eventually on the air.

What is Ethical?

It is considered unethical for a reporter to tell you exactly what the questions will be. The interview is supposed to be a spontaneous conversation. To rehearse either questions or answers is staging. But there is a fine line here.

Most reporters consider it proper to tell you the subject they're covering and broad areas they want to explore in the interview. Find out as much as you can.

Be aware that the reporter will also be sizing you up. The impression you give in those first few minutes after you connect can be critical to the questions you'll be asked, and the slant on the story.

Have Your Staff Handy

For stories that involve a lot of numbers or complicated, technical details, it's a good idea to have your staff experts nearby.

They can hand you notes or documents when you grope for the right number.

You can ask them to fetch details the reporter needs for the story. When you get the information you need, the reporter can re-ask the question. Having a friend in your corner may also make you feel more at ease and less threatened.

Don't Cram

For the interview, you don't need to do a lot of cramming. If you, the expert, and can't remember, how do you expect viewers to retain what you say? The reporter will not use many numbers in a sound bite you say on camera.

Go over the numbers before, or after, the interview. Most people can't absorb spoken statistics. They do remember analogies and perspective.

This is what we'll remember if you say in the interview:

"The money we'll spend this year treating this disease would buy everybody in the state a new Lexus."

Provide Graphs & Charts

If the audience is to retain numbers, the story will greatly benefit if it has graphs and charts that put them in perspective.

Seeing the numbers on the screen while they are spoken doubles viewer retention.

Most reporters in major cities would not think of printing or broadcasting a news release exactly as you wrote it. But they will often use your graphs or charts with no editing whatever.

Virtually every computer word processing program has graph and charting capability. Your providing graphics will help the story immensely.

Tell the reporter while you're connected by webcam that you have the graphics and can attach them to an e-mail after you hang up, if that would be helpful.

Interview Eye Contact

If the reporter were in the room with you, videotaping an interview, you'd talk to the reporter, not the camera. The camera is just listening to the conversation.

The camera doesn't ask questions. The reporter does. So if you answer into the camera, the audience reacts:

The reporter asked the question - why are you giving me the answer?

A Different Perspective

Webcam interviews have a completely different perspective. Here, you're talking to the reporter, but eye contact will depend on how the interview is going to be used.

Ask, before you begin, where they would like you to look.

If the anchor is talking to someone live, the audience knows the setup and the person being interviewed normally talks to the camera. The audience watches the interaction.

The custom is no longer rigid. Some experts are being told in their remote interviews (where the reporter was not with them when it was recorded) to look slightly to one side.

In that way, it will appear that they took part in a normal conversation, while the camera eavesdropped.

Where Do You Want Me to Look?

So ask them where they want you to look. If you don't talk to the webcam, you may be told to look slightly to one side. Keep eye contact with one edge of your monitor. They may have a choice between left or right.

Wherever they tell you to look, if your eyes get weary, take a break by looking down at your desk for a moment. As if you were in deep thought.

No Gazing Into Space

If you look off into space while you're talking or thinking about the question, the audience tends to believe you're making up the answer. That you're not being honest.

That's why placement of the webcam (learn more in the *Webcam Placement* chapter) is so critical.

Giants and Midgets

If the webcam is too high, it appears at the other end that you're being interviewed by a giant, and have to look up to maintain eye contact.

If the webcam is too low, it appears that you're the giant, looking down at this reporter who must be about four feet tall. If the webcam placement is badly done, your face will be distorted.

Try not to blink too much. That can also be interpreted as a sign of stress or deception.

Office Chair Hazards

Office chairs are a real hazard. You'll want to rock. Stress makes you twist back and forth while you rock. The chairs sometimes squeak. The viewer gets seasick as you bob up and down on screen.

A non-rocking office chair with a hydraulic lift is ideal. You can position it so the webcam is at your eye level. You can put it back to your normal working level when the interview is over.

Don't Lean Back

Sit up straight and don't lean back in the chair. Leaning back changes your body English. You tell us, without words, that you're not very enthusiastic about what you're saying.

Or that you're trying to put as much distance as you can be-

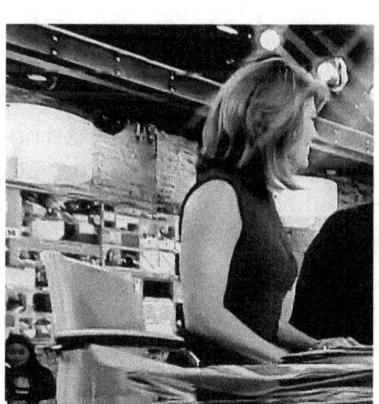

tween you and the person at the other end of the connection.

Television anchors are taught to sit this way.

Here's *CBS This Morning* anchor Norah O'Donnell (left) in a classic anchor sitting posture.

It may seem, at first, a little strange.

You move your butt to the edge of the chair. This changes your posture. It straightens the spine. You appear to be alert and self-confident.

Your words have more authority. You find that your arms on the table are lighter. It's easier to use gestures as you speak.

May Seem Awkward at First

I had to learn how to sit this way. When I do, I have to put one leg out to steady myself.

It feels like I may fall off the chair if I don't. Try it.

Everyone is different. Once you master this technique, you can do it for hours and be comfortable. It's also great if you're a witness in court, appearing on a panel, or testifying before a legislative committee.

here's a guest on that same CBS morning show. She's obviously had some on-camera training.

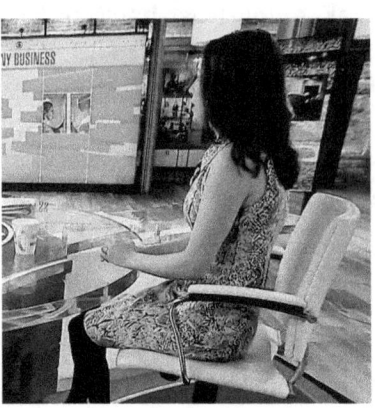

If you MUST use a swivel chair that rocks, crank the spring tension as tight as it will go. This will make the back of chair as rigid as possible. Remember not to swivel.

Take Your Time

During the interview (unless it's being broadcast live) take your time. If you start a sentence that gets tangled and confused, start again. That's what editing is for.

TV reporters also fluff their lines when they're videotaping and have to repeat them to get it right. They understand, and will almost always let you go back and start again.

If you don't understand the question, say so. If you're nervous and your mouth is dry, stop for a drink of water. Keep thinking of the living room and the friend or neighbor you imagine you're talking to. That will help relieve the nervousness.

Take More Control

Once the interview starts, most people give up all control of their lives to the reporter. Don't do that. Take more control. You can say things like:

You know, I gave you an answer several minutes ago that took me much too long to get to the point. If you'll ask me that same question again, I think I can give you a better, shorter answer. OR

I just realized I made a mistake when I answered one of your questions. What I said was not completely accurate. Let's go back over that again. I'll get it right this time.

Short and Simple

Try to talk in short, simple sentences. Lawyers and professors have a tendency to speak in outlined, organized form - firstly, secondly, thirdly - or to label their points A, B and C.

If the reporter is only interested in your third point, and you've run the words together, they may not be able to edit out "thirdly." That entire thought may be discarded in the editing process.

Other Editing Nightmares

Other common phrases like "first of all" and "as I said earlier" can create editing nightmares. There may not be enough time in a news story to let you say it twice, or to include your "first of all" point.

If you drop "as I said earlier" in the middle of a sentence, the entire sentence may have to be dumped.

Avoid dating the interview. If you say something happened yesterday, the story may not be used until tomorrow. By then whatever happened was the day before yesterday.

Like Talking to a Jury

Some of the best on-camera interviews are with trial lawyers who've spent their entire careers summing up complicated cases for jurors.

They keep it short and simple, conversational and colorful. They're good at one-sentence conclusions jurors will remember and repeat to each other in the jury room.

For the main point, they let their feelings show. Jurors are very much like those people sitting in front of the television set after a hard day's work. They're easily bored. They want it simple. They want it interesting. They want to know what it was really like to be there. How did it feel?

Beware Uhh, Ahh, You Know

It is critical that you listen to yourself speak for several minutes to learn how often you pause and say Uhh or Ahh. The entire country in recent years inserts "you know" in every other phrase. Sometimes two or three times in the same sentence.

TERRIBLE. And a very difficult habit to break.

Drop the Parentheticals

Any kind of parenthetical thought can make a sentence too long for television news. Example - a politician says:

"I've come to believe, as most of my constituents do, if they've had any experience with firearms, that every person in this country has the God-given right to own a gun."

It can be edited much easier if the politician says:

"I believe every person in this country has the God-given right to own a gun. (Pause for possible edit point)

"I'm sure most of my constituents who have any experience with firearms feel the same way I do."

With this version, the reporter can use either sentence, or both. They can also be separated to use in different parts of the story.

Anticipate the Why

Another technique that can help the editing process:

QUESTION: Then you will not vote, Senator, to outlaw Saturday Night Specials?

ANSWER: No.

QUESTION: Why?

ANSWER: The Saturday Night Special is a phony issue.

QUESTION: Why do you say that?

ANSWER: Most police officers, and most store clerks, are killed with expensive weapons. Why should the poor homeowner be denied a weapon he can afford to pro-tect himself and his family?

If you give a "Yes" or "No" answer, it will almost always be followed by "Why?"

Save Valuable Time

Anticipate the why, and if you repeat the question as part of your answer, it saves valuable response time between ques-tions and answers.

Another Way to Do It Quickly

This answer will enable the reporter to cram the entire re-sponse into about two-thirds as much time:

> QUESTION: Then you will not vote, Senator, to outlaw Saturday Night Specials?

> ANSWER: I will never vote to outlaw Saturday Night Specials. They're a phony issue. Most police officers ... etc.

Incorporating the question into your answer allows the re-porter to drop the sound bite into the story without having to set up what you were asked.

Show Me While You Tell Me

What the audience sees, if you're genuine, may communi-cate more than what they hear. Years ago, advertising agencies learned how to use visual suggestions in print.

A lot can be said in a picture that doesn't require words. Be-cause of television's time limitations, that technique has be-come a science.

The real message is visual, not verbal. And it is usually more powerful than words.

How TV Commercials Use Visuals

Luxury car commercials tell us about the wonderful engi-neering or handling of the automobile. But the more effective message is what we see.

The driver is pulling up to a home that cost several million dollars. Or sliding behind the wheel at the country club. Or at the airport, with a corporate jet in the background.

And, of course, there is a trophy wife or husband in the passenger seat. The key visual message: If you're rich, sophisticated, influential, sexually attractive, you'll buy this car.

Visual Shorthand

Politicians have learned to use the same kind of visual symbolism to communicate with their constituents. After a flood or earthquake, it is now a tribal ritual for the governor to survey the damage from a National Guard helicopter.

Is that really necessary? Can't governors get reports from experts who are better equipped to assess the damage?

Yes, but we've come to expect a personal visit. If we don't see the governor, the president or the vice president at the scene of a major disaster, we think they don't care.

This used to be called a "photo opportunity." The new word for it is "optics."

More Important Than What You Say

I have done a lot of law enforcement training. Chiefs and sheriffs worry about what they will say the day an officer is killed in the line of duty.

I tell them I'm much more concerned about what the public will SEE them doing. A picture is worth a thousand words. Maybe a million.

You need to be seen at the scene, I tell them. You know TV cameras will be at the hospital, at the officer's home. And if you're not at the funeral, kiss your job good-bye. Being there speaks volumes. Not being there also delivers a powerful message.

Clothing Messages

The clothes you wear are part of the visual shorthand. When he was president, Jimmy Carter liked to be interviewed in a plaid shirt and sweater.

To enhance his "just plain folks" image, Carter often carried a piece of luggage when he was embarking from a plane or helicopter - even though a small army of aides and Secret Service agents were there, empty-handed. Richard Nixon wanted to suggest a more regal kind of presidency. You sometimes wondered if he slept in a coat and tie.

Barack Obama was the master of knowing when to get rid of his coat, and sometimes his tie. It depends on the time and place where you'll be filmed.

> (An aside - Almost nobody shoots film any more. Filming (the verb) has taken on the meaning of any video which is shot. Partly because there are so many different kinds of recording media now.)

Coats and Ties

A CEO wearing his coat and tie behind an immaculate desk tells us, subliminally, that he is a figurehead who is aloof, unfamiliar with his employees, and rarely gets involved in the nuts and bolts of running the company. A paper shuffler.

Let's design another scenario. The desktop has some papers scattered on it, with a computer at one side. The CEO has his coat off, tie loose, sleeves rolled up. The impression changes. He seems hands-on, hard-working, personally involved.

Learn From Candidates

You can learn a lot from presidential candidates. They have very high-priced consultants who tell them what to wear. During his 2008 and 2012 campaigns, Barack Obama usually appeared with a dress shirt, no coat, no tie.

After he was elected, he did the same thing when he went on the road to sell his issues. But for recorded messages from the Oval Office, he wore a coat and tie.

As this is being written, Donald Trump does not seem yet to have figured this out.

I suggest to my clients that if they normally come to work in business clothes, they should also keep some more casual clothes at the office, for certain unexpected interviews.

There is now a demeaning term for men who wear coats and ties - "the suits." Most Americans no longer dress like that at work. The message you deliver in that kind of clothing may be that you're old, out-of-date, and uninvolved in the real work your organization does.

What Should Women Wear?

Women's clothing is much more complex. There are so many more choices. The standard coat and tie for men is a sort of uniform. As both a public official and candidate, Hillary Clinton decided to wear a pant suit, no matter what the occasion.

It was partly to hide the weight she gained as she aged. But after a while, her clothing reminded me of the uniforms Asian leaders adopted.

If she had asked for my advice (she didn't) I would have suggested that her failure to wear different styles might make some people suspect she was inflexible in her thinking or personality.

More Suggestions for Women

This may seem obvious, but wear something that fits. It shouldn't sag or bag. Clothes that are too tight, or tug at your waist or chest, really stand out and catch the viewers' attention.

Don't wear something that's too big, either. The color of clothes, or the style, matters less than how it fits.

That said, don't wear colors that are too loud or bright. They distract. If you have time to choose, select items that complement your face color.

Makeup Ideas

Make sure lipstick and blush match and don't clash. For most women, matte finish lipstick works better than gloss. Be sure to use powder on any spots that tend to be shiny.

Use light-colored eye shadow directly over your lids, darker colors in the lid crease, light skin color tones under the eyebrows, and apply moderate to heavy eyeliner and mascara.

Do a dress rehearsal with your clothes. Wear them and make a test recording with your webcam. Clothes that fit well when you stand may do strange and unusual things when you're sitting.

Jewelry and Accessories

Earrings should be no larger than a quarter, and not dangle or swing. Most necklaces tend to be gorgeous in person, but if we start looking at it while you're talking, we may miss the essence of your brief comments. If you wear neck jewelry, make sure it has a non-reflective finish.

Solution for a Man's Bald Spot

In webcam interviews, there will usually be an overhead light that glares on a man's oily bald spot(s). Before the interview, wipe those areas with rubbing alcohol. It will eliminate the glare.

In Early TV, Blue Was White

In the early days of television news, men were told to wear light blue shirts. That's because they were shooting black-and-white film. A white shirt glowed in the harsh light and high-contrast film. A blue shirt looked white.

With today's color cameras, white looks white, and blue looks blue.

But the automatic sensor in today's cameras reads the general light level coming through the lens. Light clothing makes the aperture of the camera lens constrict, just as the iris in the human eye does. Dark clothing does the opposite (more on this in the *Lighting and Background* chapter).

Generally, your clothes for television should be subdued. Plain, solid colors are best. Stay away from stripes, checks and bold prints. The electronics in modern video cameras can make patterns seem to ripple and pulsate. Make the clothes fit the story.

My simple rule for both genders: If we remember what you were wearing, you wore the wrong thing.

Don't Get a Haircut

If you know a webcam interview is imminent, don't go to the beauty salon or the barber shop. We will probably be able to tell that you spruced up for the interview.

Remember, this is supposedly a spontaneous, unrehearsed conversation, not a formal portrait or glamour shoot.

I was fairly new to television when I covered the 1972 Republican National Convention in Miami Beach. There was a demonstration where the crowd became violent and police used teargas.

Effects of Teargas

I do not do teargas well. I get wheezy and my eyes get terribly irritated. I've been temporarily blinded by teargas.

On that night in 1972, I ran to the apartment WPLG had rented as a studio, across from the Convention Center. I told them what was happening in the street. In addition to my red, teary eyes, I was drenched with sweat.

"Get in the chair," a producer told me. "We'll do a live cut-in."

"Let me wash my face and comb my hair," I said.

"No, no, no," the producer said. "You look like shit. That will tell us more than anything you're gonna say."

I was beginning to understand TV reporting, and its old saying: DON'T TELL US. SHOW US.

Wear Your Eyeglasses

If you normally wear eyeglasses, wear them for the interview. Without them, your eyes will have to work harder. You'll squint. There will be a crease through a man's sideburns and depressions in your nose where the glasses were before the interview.

But Not Sunglasses

But don't wear dark glasses for webcam interviews. In this culture, you're supposed to look people in the eye when you talk to them. The stereotyped movie hoodlum wears dark glasses during conversations - perhaps to hide the evil thoughts his eyes would reveal if we could see them.

Beware - glasses that darken in sunlight might also turn dark if you've set up auxiliary lighting for your webcam.

If you're going to do a lot of television interviews, have your optician treat your eyeglass lenses with the invisible, anti-reflective coating that television reporters and anchors use. It's very much like the coating on a camera lens.

Reading the Details

Normally, I advise clients to NEVER read speeches or statements. Unless you've worked in broadcasting, you don't read well. It seems canned and insincere.

But there is an exception.

As a television reporter, I developed a technique for live re-motes that let me read exact words from an important doc-ument. It added authority and credibility.

If three legislators had been indicted for bribery, I'd do the live standup in front of the courthouse, with the indictment in my hand.

"Let Me Read It to You"

Off-the-cuff, I'd summarize what had happened, then say, "Let me read to you what the grand jury found."

I'd have a paragraph high-lighted. I'd read it, then continue in my own words until I reached another section where I wanted to use exactly what the grand jury reported.

You can use the same technique in a webcam interview.

Stilted Phrases You'd Never Speak

You will be much more effective in a webcam interview if you use words and phrases you'd use in normal conversa-tion. I'd like the people watching the interview to say to themselves: Did he/she know this was being recorded?

I hate interviews where the guy on camera says, "I cannot comprehend the significance of these occurrences."

I think he means, "I have no idea what's going on here."

Or the woman who says, "I proceeded into the premises and was immediately impressed by the proliferation of styles."

I think she said "When I went into that store, I was blown away by the variety of stuff they sell."

Gestures and Animation

In normal conversation, people gesture with their hands. They have facial animation. A raised eyebrow. A frown. They shake their heads to emphasize something they disapprove of. They lean forward to emphasize a comment. It becomes a physical exclamation point.

And they pause. . . .

To let the idea sink in. . . .

The half-second pause is a WONDERFUL ingredient for news media interviews. It gives the listener time to digest what you've just said.

It also provides an easy editing point.

Creating Sound Bites

I estimate that about 35,000 people are interviewed by the news media in America every day. This is hard to believe, but I already know exactly what the reporters are going to ask in about 90 per cent of those interviews.

It doesn't matter where the interview takes place. Doesn't matter who the reporter is - who is being interviewed - doesn't even matter what the story is about. I know the key question:

How Do You Feel . . .?

In virtually every news interview, the reporter will ask how you feel about something.

The perennial question has been institutionalized by a TV news story formula - the Sony Sandwich. It has spread to all news media.

Disguising the Question

Reporters are so aware of their trite question, they try to disguise it. But it is still the search for the human perspective.

- Tell me - what you were thinking, just before the plane hit the water?

- When the officer walked in with your baby in his arms, what was it like?

- What was your reaction when you become aware you had been bilked by your financial advisor?

- Did you think you were going to die?

Someday, we may go through that same experience. We want to know how it feels to do what you did ... see what you saw ... hear what you heard.

What Was It Like to Be There?

How do you feel is usually asking, "What was it like to be there?" That has always been the essence of storytelling. I want to hear from survivors of a mass shooting incident their inner thoughts as it unfolded. I may someday be caught in a similar situation. I'd like to plan a way to survive.

Tell me the story of a blind child who can see for the first time, and I get a lump in my throat.

When she tells me what she's feeling, I may cry.

The Human Perspective

Interviews inject the human perspective in news stories. Few people outside the news media understand this basic purpose for the "feeling" question that will elicit the quote or the sound bite the storyteller is looking for.

It is sandwiched between the facts the reporter gives at the beginning, and the conclusion drawn at the end.

Building the Sony Sandwich

Standup Close

The Interview is the meat of the sandwich

Opening Summary, Voice Over

The Sony Sandwich Formula

Something you say during your webcam interview with a TV reporter will become the meat in a Sony Sandwich - the "sound bite."

It gives the story warmth and personality, emotion and flavor, color and dimension.

If it's a network story, they rarely use more than 10 seconds from an interview. A local station may let you speak a few seconds longer. This story formula is sometimes called a "package."

The beginning of the Sony Sandwich is the bottom half of the bun. The reporter quickly sketches the scenario. It is a summary of the story. Sometimes only a sentence or two.

We frequently have not seen the reporter yet.

The Voice-Over Summary

The summary is delivered V/O (voice/over) while we are shown video of the place or event the story is about. After the reporter has set up the basic facts, we go to a central figure in the story.

The Key Question

That person is asked something like:

- How did you feel when you learned your son was alive?

- (On election night) How does it feel to lose after 24 years in the Senate?

- How does it feel to win the lottery?

- How do you feel about the President's proposal?

- How do you feel, now that your company has gone bankrupt?

- Do you feel this proposal is necessary?

Topping off the Sandwich

And then the reporter closes out the story. Often with a standup, looking into the camera, in front of the spot the story is about. The reporter summarizes, telling us what to expect next. Here's the formula closing:

What Does it All Mean?

What does it all mean? Only time will tell. I'm Tom Trite, Channel Four, Action News.

People in certain professions are interviewed more often than others. The ones who get the hang of it find reporters coming back to them on future stories. They make the reporter's job so much easier. Unfortunately, some careers tend to create poor prospects for interviews.

Career Influence On Camera Style

Doctors, lawyers, scientists and accountants are often terrible on camera. They speak their own, professional jargon, as though we, too, had Ph.Ds in their specialty. They provide dry, lengthy, logical, step-by-step reasoning, with lots of footnotes. The subject matter is complicated. The simplest question takes three minutes to answer.

This kind of interview is a horror to edit. The people interviewed call the next day to complain that they were quoted out of context. On camera, they often sound like robotic voice synthesizers. They've been conditioned to talk that way by writing too many reports, reading too many articles written by colleagues, and by testifying in court.

Human Synthesizers

The cop who just caught two armed robbers after a shootout speaks very normally until the camera comes. Then he says:

> My unit was dispatched to 4481 Ocean Street at nineteen hundred hours. As I approached, Code Three, I observed two white males rapidly exiting the dispatched location in an easterly direction with weapons drawn. When the perpetrators observed my vehicle, they commenced firing. One projectile impacted my vehicle. I then returned fire.

What Did He Say?

What did he say? I think he said:

"As I rolled up, these two guys with guns were running out of the jewelry store. They saw the patrol car and started shooting. When the first bullet hit my windshield, I jumped out and shot back." Which leads to the reporter's question:

"You ever been shot at before?"

"Nope."

"How did it feel?"

"Scared the hell out of me."

You can probably guess which section of the interview is certain to be included in the Sony Sandwich.

What Are We Afraid Of?

Survey after survey has shown that stage fright is America's biggest fear. Bigger than war, cancer, divorce, dying in a plane or car crash. What are we so afraid of onstage?

I think we're afraid of looking stupid.

People in front of a camera often talk non-conversation because they're afraid they'll make a mistake and look dumb.

What Will the Boss Think?

They're not sure the boss will like the idea of their talking to a TV reporter.

So they cram and memorize, to avoid mistakes. They want to be walking, infallible encyclopedias. But they're boring, and we don't even listen.

Becoming What You Most Fear

Applicants being interviewed by webcam for a job often do the same thing. They can look like stupid drones. Robots with a recorded message. The one thing they most fear.

Other people deal with on-camera stress by drawing themselves into tight little knots, making their voices small and flat, as they say every word very carefully.

They pause a lot. On TV, they are deadly. More than five seconds, and everybody in the audience will be snoring.

The Original Story Formula

The Sony Sandwich evolved from the original American news story formula - developed by newspapers in the 1800s - the Inverted Pyramid.

At the beginning of the story - into the first paragraph, if possible - the reporter tried to cram all the important facts. Who, What, When, Where, Why.

From that broad beginning, the story narrowed down to a point at the bottom where unimportant details were thrown in. Pure trivia.

The inverted pyramid had several practical purposes. Correspondents in faraway places (St. Louis was the edge of civilization in those days) sent their stories to New York or Washington by telegraph.

The Telegraph was Unreliable

The telegraph was not very reliable. So if it failed sometime during transmission, the home office would at least have the important stuff. If the entire story reached the newspaper, readers knew they could drop off in mid-story and not miss anything critical.

In those days, newspaper stories were set in lead type. Down in the composing room, they had to fit each line of type into a page form before the newspaper went to press.

If the type didn't fit, the employees in the composing room were told to cut from the bottom until it did fit.

Throwing Away Paragraphs

Just throw away the last paragraph, they were told. Maybe the last two paragraphs. There were barrels where the lead type was thrown to be recycled.

The typesetters were not editors. They were craftsmen. As a result, stories sometimes seemed to have been edited with a chain saw.

The Sandwich Spreads

Because the Sony Sandwich works so well, both radio and newspapers adopted it for their own use. Understanding the formula will help you craft a quote that will be used exactly as you said it - without editing - in newspapers, radio, TV, or Internet podcasts.

Avoiding Misquotes

If you can learn to do this, you'll seldom be misquoted or taken out of context. You'll find your interviews go very quickly. As soon as reporters hear the magic, formula quote, they tell you goodbye.

And they'll ask you for more webcam interviews in the future for stories in your area of expertise.

The FACE Formula

I invented the FACE Formula to help you remember what kind of quote the reporter is looking for.

If you're the subject of the interview, and we're going to see your face on TV. Keep these factors in mind:

F eelings

A nalysis

C ompelling C's

E nergy

Let's look at each factor in the formula:

Feelings

Let the audience know what you're feeling. Go back from time to time and review the Sony Sandwich formula to help you reflexively craft quotes that begin with how you feel.

That first phrase sets us up to receive your reasons for feeling that way. Like:

"I'm really angry about this."

Or sad, happy, encouraged, disappointed, afraid, surprised, confident ... You get the idea.

Analysis

Give them your assessment of the situation. In one phrase or sentence, tell them what the bottom line is. The audience wants your expert opinion on the subject. That's why the reporter is talking to you.

But to avoid the cutting room floor, the expert must be able to translate into everyday language. Analysis interviews often deal with statistics.

Numbers Must Have Perspective

If you use numbers, they are meaningless unless you put the numbers in perspective.

Many experts speak in strange tongues.

After the reporter has said that experts claim there is no danger from the accident within the nuclear power plant, we see an interview with an internationally recognized scientist.

He says on camera:

> *We've put the effluent through exhaustive electron microscopy plus radiofluorocarbon laser analysis and we come up with a count of point four, seven, zero micro-mini roentgens.*

What did he say?

Translation, Please

Translated, I think he said: You'd get more radiation sitting in front of a TV for two hours than you would if you took a bath in the water that leaked out.

The Compelling C's

Most news stories revolve around at least one of these basic elements. Notice the underlined feeling words:

Catastrophe - "I'm afraid we're facing a global disaster if we don't change the way we dispose of toxic waste. And I'm surprised by those who refuse to believe the evidence."

Crisis - "I'm astounded by their stupidity. The tidal surge will sweep across the highway and cut off their escape route if they don't leave now."

Conflict - "I hate him and everything he stands for. I'll fight him to my last breath."

Change - "I'm confident things are going to be different around here after the election, when we win control of the Legislature."

Crime and Corruption - "I grieve for my father. He was such a good man. And I will not rest until they catch who did this."

Color - (They used to call it human interest.) "I'm really amused. Anyone who believes that also believes thunder curdles milk."

Celebrities - "I'm awed by his technical skill. He can manipulate that computer the way Michael Jordan controls a basketball."

Energy

There is one major difference in talking on camera and talking to your friends in their living room. To be effective on camera, your conversation needs to project energy.

Onscreen, you will ALWAYS be more boring than you are in real life.

Like a salesperson who must believe in the product, you must show that you truly believe what you're saying.

Since so many stories for television news involve conflict and imminent danger, you must convince us - through the energy you invest in what you're saying - that we ought to be concerned, too.

Executive Cool = Dull

Some executives in high-pressure jobs adopt a cool, clinical personality that says to their employees, "I know exactly what I'm doing. If the building were on fire, I would lead you to safety and save your life." That deliberate, slow, calculating style can appear, - on TV - to be boredom, disinterest, or a mask for insecurity.

You Need to See and Hear Yourself

I constantly tell my clients that they need to see themselves on camera to know what they really look like. In our minds, we have imbedded high school yearbook photos of ourselves. That image distorts our perception of ourselves.

The mirror lies. The person I see when I shave is about 20 years younger, 20 pounds lighter than the person on my webcam screen.

A webcam is an ideal learning tool. You can record practice interviews and replay them instantly until you're happy with the results.

The Boring Phenomenon

Be aware that there is a major distortion when we watch interviews on television or a computer monitor. Time slows down. You may not catch this as you watch your own performance. But others will.

Unless you inject energy into what you say, our perception of the person on screen is that you are incredibly dull and boring.

The Slow Motion Experience

Why does that happen? I think I have the answer. Have you ever been in a life-threatening crisis where everything seemed to go into slow motion?

I've questioned thousands of people in my workshops about these experiences. It seems to be universal.

In the moments before the car crash, they watched the on-coming car spinning gracefully, edging closer, as they carefully analyzed whether it would hit them.

Life-Threatening Crises

A pilot told about losing an engine on takeoff. It seemed to take half a day to turn the plane and get it back on the runway.

A scuba diver in a cave ran out of air and made a desperate attempt to reach the surface. He lost consciousness, and would have drowned. But he was rescued by his buddies and resuscitated. He said the time he was struggling to reach the surface before he blacked out was only a few seconds. But it seemed more like hours.

A woman thrown up through her car's sunroof when it rolled over said she felt like she was hovering in mid-air, watching her car turning slowly below her.

Shooting As He Fell

A cop was shot at close range. The bullet knocked him on his back. As he fell, he was able to pull his pistol and fire three times before he hit the ground.

It was easy to do, he said, because it seemed like he was suspended in mid-air for about five minutes. He said he even had time to aim the shot that hit his assailant in the chest.

The technical name for the phenomenon is tachypsychia. Part of it is caused by the sudden dump of adrenaline into your bloodstream. The other factor is your total focus on what is happening.

Our Perception Changes Time

It is my theory that when we watch an interview on a computer monitor or television screen, we are focused just enough to change our perception of time.

I see this happen regularly in my seminars. I videotape an interview and then we have instant replay. The person who seemed to be speaking in a normal voice just a few seconds ago now seems to have lost energy and conviction.

I know the replay is accurate. It is our perception as we focus that robs the interview of its energy and passion.

By practicing with recorded webcam interviews, you can study yourself. You can learn to inject just the right amount of energy to make our perception of you on the screen match what we would see in real life.

Don't Overdo It

Just don't overdo it, so you seem shrill or obsessed. There is a different line for everyone. And a gender gap between how we perceive men and women. Only practice will find that line.

Forget About Memorizing

In preparing for a webcam interview, don't memorize or write out a script. It makes the interview seem staged and rehearsed.

I recommend that before the interview, you go over in your mind the main points you'd like to include. You need to have that central theme in your head, and some sub-sections that connect to that central idea. No more than three.

If you're afraid the stress of the interview will make you forget, write yourself a cheat sheet, the same way students cheat on exams.

Using a Cheat Sheet

The cheat sheet should be one-word cues - bullet points - that will refresh your memory if your mind goes blank.

Put the cheat sheet where you can glance down and see it But ONLY IF YOU NEED TO.

The trick is to look thoughtful, pause and glance down as if you're thinking deeply, then look back at the camera to finish the thought.

This is a natural head movement in normal conversation. Be careful about setting up a rhythm of repeatedly looking down and then back at the webcam. If you do that, we'll know you're reading.

Nobody will know you cheated if you do it right.

A Psychological Crutch

Just writing the key points will help you remember. Having the cheat sheet handy is an assuring psychological crutch. If it's there, you probably won't need it.

Remember - you have to condense, condense, condense. In public speaking courses, the instructor gives you a subject and forces you to make an immediate, extemporaneous talk. The exercise teaches you to think and talk on your feet.

Some Training Exercises

To train yourself for webcam interviews, try to say how you feel about a difficult topic - and three reasons why you feel that way - in 12 seconds or less.

Pick tough, complicated subjects and practice with a video camera. In one sentence, say how you feel - and why - about difficult subjects like:

- Legalized abortion
- Gun control
- Capital punishment
- Prayer in schools
- Ethnic job quotas
- Illegal immigration
- Taxes and government spending

There is no quick miracle drug, no magic diet, no futuristic machine to make you an instant success. It takes tough, conscientious mental calisthenics to be truly good at it.

This exercise, practiced regularly, will develop your mental agility for condensing what you know and feel about complicated subjects.

Congressional Pros

The real pros are congressional leaders who've been interviewed several times a day for 20 years. They develop stopwatches in their heads. Before the camera rolls, they discuss the story with the reporter. They get some idea of how their quotes will be used.

The Quickie Interview

"How much time do you need?" the senator asks, clearing his throat and brushing his hair aside.

"About 12 seconds," the reporter tells him.

"OK. I'm ready."

"Rolling."

The senator speaks for 12 seconds. Perhaps 11. Sometimes, 13. And then he stops. He has learned the language, and the game. He edits himself. There can be no distortion. He is rarely quoted out of context. The entire process has taken less than five minutes.

You Can Do It, Too

Most of those who've learned to speak in sound bites did it the hard way, through trial and error. For many, it became a self-defense tactic. The news media are kinder to some people than others.

One person's slip is never aired. Another, similar stumble becomes the comedy element in tonight's news.

Learn From Others' Mistakes

Watch and listen to interviews on TV newcasts. Make notes on the people who are effective. Learn from the mistakes and blunders of other people.

If you can learn how to speak media language, and give a formula response to the formula question, you almost guarantee they'll use what you said, exactly as you said it.

With no editing, misquoting or taking out of context.

You're the Expert

Often, the person being interviewed is an authority, whose assessment of the situation is important to our understanding it. In court testimony, witnesses are not allowed to express their opinions or feelings. Unless they are certified as expert witnesses. Only then they can tell the jury how they feel about the evidence.

When you become the subject of a media interview, it's often because you're the expert witness who can put things in perspective. When reporters ask experts how they feel, they're really asking for opinion or analysis.

Verbal Shorthand

Words that express feeling tell us a lot very quickly. They are verbal shorthand - headline words that communicate like no others in our language. They get to the heart of the story, and set us up to hear your reasons for feeling that way.

When the reporter asks how you feel about something, it can mean, "What do you think about this? - What is your reaction to the situation? - What is your opinion?" But we will understand your reaction - your opinion - your conclusion - much more clearly if you tell us how you FEEL.

News stories are so formularized, it is almost a paint-by-numbers process. I've collected a list of words, from which at least one will fit virtually any news interview in which you're asked that key question. Take your pick.

Words That Say How You Feel

A Abandoned, Abused, Afraid, Aggravated, Alienated, Alone, Amazed, Ambushed, Amused, Angry, Anxious, Ashamed, Astonished, Astounded

B Bamboozled, Banged up, Battered, Bedazzled, Besieged, Betrayed, Blessed, Blinded, Bored, Bothered, Broken, Burned out

C Caught in the middle, Cautious, Certain, Challenged, Chagrined, Cheated, Concerned, Confident, Conflicted, Confused, Conned, Crazy

D Dazzled, Deceived, Delighted, Deserted, Disappointed, Dismayed, Disorganized, Distraught, Distressed, Doubtful

E Ecstatic, Elated Embarrassed, Encouraged, Energized, Enthusiastic, Envious, Excited, Exhausted, Exposed

F Fearful, Fed up, Forgiven, Forgiving, Frantic, Free, Friendly, Frightened, Frustrated, Fenced in

G Glad, Glorious, Grateful, Gratified, Great! Grief-stricken, Guilty, Gullible, Gutted

H Happy, Harried, Hate (I hate it!), Haunted, Helpless, High, Hobbled, Hollow, Homicidal, Honored, Hoodwinked, Hopeful, Hopeless, Horrendous, Horrible, Horrified, Hounded, Humble, Humiliated, Hungry, Hurt

I Impatient, Impotent, Ineffective, Insecure, Inspired, Insulted, Intrigued, Invaded, Irritated, Isolated

J Jaded, Jealous, Jilted, Jinxed, Jolted, Joyful, Jubilant, Justified

L Livid, Lonely, Love (I love it!), Loser (Like a loser), Lucky, Lively

M Mad, Maligned, Marvelous, Misguided, Misunderstood, Mortified, Mystified

N Naked, Nauseated, Neglected, Negligent, Nostalgic, Nurtured

O Offended, On top of the world, Optimistic, Out of touch, Outgunned, Outnumbered, Outraged, Overjoyed, Overwhelmed

P Paranoid, Parental, Peeved, Pessimistic, Pleased, Powerful, Powerless, Proud, Put down, Put out, Puzzled

R Ready, Recharged Regretful, Reinforced, Rejoice, Rejuvenated, Relieved, Reminiscent, Resentful, Responsive, Rested

S Sad, Safe, Sated, Satisfied, Saturated, Scared, Secure, Shocked, Shunned, Sick, Skeptical, Sorry, Stupid, Support-ive, Sure, Surprised, Surrounded, Swindled, Sympathetic, Shaken

T Targeted, Terrible, Terrific, Terrified, Tired, Torn, Tram-pled, Traumatized

U Uncertain, Undaunted, Under control, Underwhelmed, Undone, Unforgiving, Unjustly accused, Unsatisfied, Un-wanted, Unworthy, Used

V Victimized, Victorious, Vulnerable

W Warm, Weak, Weary, Weepy, Winner (Like a winner), Wonderful, Worried, Worn out, Wounded

Condition Words

Some of the feeling words in the list above are not real feel-ings. They are conditions that convey several emotions or strong feelings.

When you say, "I feel betrayed," you tell us - with just one word - that you feel angry, deceived, abandoned, vulnerable. If you feel surrounded, you are feeling insecure, outnum-bered, overwhelmed.

Interviews add flavor and spice to a story. Once the conflict, the catastrophe, the crisis is established, we want to hear the participants. We want to know how they feel about it. Their reaction to it.

Guaranteed- Sound Bites

Sound bites they'll use for sure:

- "I'm embarrassed. The mayor has made a terrible mistake."

- "It's frightening. This guy is completely bonkers. He'll take us back to the Stone Age."

- "I wasn't afraid - I was just terribly sad, that I'd never see my son again."

- "Fantastic. After the surgery, I feel like a kid again."

A Word of Caution:

There are a few rare times when showing too much emotion on camera can be hazardous to your career. We don't expect a homicide detective to break down at a murder scene. Unless the victim is his partner, or his own child.

Some history: Edmund Muskie may have lost his campaign for the Democratic presidential nomination in 1972 when he became teary during a speech in the snow in New Hampshire. He was defending his wife after a newspaper editorial defamed her. In those days, Americans thought that made him appear weak.

The Rules Began to Change

But then society's expectations began to change. During the televised 1988 presidential debates, Democratic nominee Gov. Michael Dukakis - an opponent of capital punishment - was asked how he would feel on that issue if his wife was a rape or murder victim.

Dukakis showed no emotion. His answer was academic, distant, unfeeling. People in the audience thought: What sort of man is this, who doesn't react to his wife being violated or killed? His nickname became "Zorba the accountant." He did not win

A Kinder, Gentler President

In that same campaign, George H. W. Bush's media experts asked focus groups what kind of President they wanted. Based on that research, Bush promised to be a "kinder, gentler President."

In television interviews, Bush began to talk about his family as sensitive, caring people. The Bushes, he said, show what they feel, and sometimes the men are not afraid to cry.

Schwarzkopf's Tears

One of the most dramatic demonstrations of how the rules were changing came three years later. Barbara Walters interviewed Army Gen. Norman Schwarzkopf in Saudi Arabia for _20/20_. It was 1991, shortly after the Persian Gulf War ended. Schwarzkopf had been the commanding general in that war.

"Stormin' Norman" talked about how much he missed his family, half a world away, and the tears welled in his eyes. When Walters asked about his dead father, who had also been a general, the tears came again. "I'm sure he'd be proud of me," Schwarzkopf said, his lower lip trembling.

Generals Don't Cry

There was a long pause in the interview. "You know," Walters said, "The old picture of generals - is that generals don't cry."

"Sure they do," Schwarzkopf shot back, naming Civil War generals Ulysses Grant and William Tecumseh Sherman.

"And these were the tough old guys. Lee cried at the loss of human life, the pressures that were brought to bear. Lincoln cried. Frankly, any man that doesn't cry scares me a little bit.

"I don't think I would like a man who was incapable of enough emotion to get tears in his eyes every now and then. That's not a human being."

September 11, 2001

A sea change of attitude about showing emotion in America came 10 years later, after the terrorist attacks of Sept. 11, 2001. Police officers, firefighters, and reporters wept openly on television as the news media covered the carnage and its aftermath.

And so did those watching the story unfold. Americans became more human, more able to express their caring and their grief.

Howard Dean's Scream

As I said earlier, you need to see yourself on camera to know where the emotional line is for you. Remember Howard Dean's candidacy to be the Democratic nominee for President in 2004?

He became so overly enthusiastic at a rally after the Iowa caucuses, some voters felt he really didn't have the demeanor to be President.

Obama's Failure to Show Emotion

As President Barack Obama struggled with the economic recession, health care and two wars after he took office in 2009, his public approval ratings began to plummet. His cold, intellectual way of dealing with major issues made people feel he was distant and uncaring.

Not until the incumbent Democrats in Congress were trounced in the November, 2010 elections did Obama go back to the enthusiastic style he had displayed when he was running for election.

Mitt Romney's Lukewarm Support

In the 2012 presidential campaign, analysts struggled to figure out why Republicans were lukewarm about Mitt Romney. The best guess was that his life of privilege and wealth had conditioned him to not care about those with less wealth, and to be protective about his private life and his inner feelings.

That gave many in the middle class a concern that he was not one of them. That he did not react to life as they did. That he would not make critical decisions the way they would.

Sandy Hook Murders

And then another watershed event occurred. Twenty-six teachers and first-graders were killed in a mass murder at Sandy Hook Elementary School in December, 2012.

Barrack Obama, many reporters, anchor people and police officers wept on camera as they talked about the slaughtered children.

And viewers, choked up in their living rooms, felt it was perfectly OK for the journalists and first responders to show their feelings, too.

Gender Conflicts

There are also gender conflicts in the culture. In their childhood, men who are now middle-aged or older were taught not to show their feelings. Men don't cry, they were told. Men don't show fear, or pain.

Women are caught in a crossfire as the culture shifts. Cry at the office and the men in power are likely to invoke the old standards that said showing emotion was a sign of weakness.

"Just like a woman," they mutter under their breath.

America still has many double standards for men and women. An angry, determined man is called aggressive. Bold.

An angry woman may be called shrill. Bitchy. Emotionally unstable. Hormonally challenged.

That's why seeing yourself on video is so important. Everybody has a different threshold in expressing how you feel without appearing to go overboard.

Show Your Humanity

I'm not suggesting that you cry in every interview. My goal for you is to show your humanity. If you do, those quotes will be used, and used exactly as you spoke them. In context. No misquotes.

The formula that reporters use is so predictable, I make a bet with my seminar groups: Send me a transcript of your next media interview. Print, radio, television. Doesn't matter. I'll buy you dinner if I can't pick the quote or sound bite the reporter used when the story was printed or broadcast.

It will always be the quote that tells us how you feel. I've made the bet with more than 100,000 people, and I've never lost.

Think of Your Audience

Listening to one end of a telephone conversation, you can usually tell who's on the other end. If it's long distance, most people tend to talk louder.

Subconsciously, they think they have to speak up to be heard clearly a thousand miles away. For some reason I can't figure out, we also seem to talk louder on a cell phone call.

We slow down if we sense that the person at the other end of the line is old, or has a foreign accent. We change the tone of our voice if we're talking to a child, or a lover. The same kind of subtle changes take place when people talk in front of cameras and microphones.

An Audience of One or Two

If they know the mic is hot, many people reflexively talk as if they're making a speech in a huge auditorium. There may be half a million people - perhaps more - out there listening. With a crowd that large, you subconsciously make sure the people in the back row hear what you have to say.

But they're not in one, humongous auditorium.

The video audience is one or two people. It is Joe Sixpack and Aunt Millie, sitting in the living room or kitchen, six or eight feet from the TV set. It is one person, watching a podcast on a computer monitor 18 inches away.

One of the secrets of video interviews is to keep that tiny audience of one or two people in mind.

Think of Someone Else

If the person on your webcam screen is a famous TV personality, or a doctor, it may help you to imagine you're talking to someone else. Someone you know well. Your spouse, a neighbor, the cashier at the restaurant where you have lunch.

In your mind, you're talking to one of them, not the reporter, anchorperson or doctor.

Mind-Set & Body Language

Changing your mind-set will change your body language. In the noise and confusion of a political rally, a candidate holds up his arms and flashes a big grin to communicate warmth and charm as he tries to woo the crowd.

He uses a very different kind of smile and body language later that night if he's trying to seduce a beautiful woman sitting across the table from him in a quiet restaurant.

You Don't Need to Project

If you think of a large audience, you will instinctively project your voice to reach them. You don't need to do that. But it takes a lot of practice to squelch that natural inclination. Today's microphones are so sensitive they can pick up a whisper across a room.

For video interviews, the most powerful message is delivered with a whispered shout. It is emotional emphasis and intensity - not loudness - that will get your point across most effectively.

Clinton's Town Meetings

Former President Bill Clinton's best style for TV has always been town hall meetings. He was at his best talking to a specific person, not the entire crowd. He still is.

Focusing On Just One Person

He takes a step or two toward the person who asks a question. He maintains intense eye contact to enhance our perception that he is totally absorbed in this very personal conversation with someone whose opinion matters. We like that about famous people.

Remember, the camera is not one of your professional colleagues. It's somebody you just met at a dinner party, who knows absolutely nothing about your job and won't understand its jargon.

The Camera Spots Phonies

The camera detects phonies. Bring to the conversation the real person inside you, not a front. Let your emotions show, if they're real. You can be angry, or sad, pleased with yourself or your organization, shocked or dismayed at what you've just learned.

The reporter will not use many facts or figures when your sound bite is chosen to include in the story. Nor your recitation of the facts. There is not enough time. You probably don't have the skill to boil down the facts extemporaneously.

Writing Short Takes a Long Time

Even experienced reporters have trouble doing that.

To condense them to 10 or 15 seconds can require a half-hour at the keyboard, eliminating a word, rewriting a phrase to save another few seconds.

A famous quote, attributed to several people: "I'm writing you a long letter because I didn't have time to write a short one."

Tell Me a Story

Another important way to persuade the reporter that you know what you're talking about - or to reinforce your position - is to make a statement and then tell a story that illustrates that statement. Transitions like:

We MUST do something about the way we care for wounded veterans. Just yesterday, I was at the local veterans' hospital and talked with a man who ...

Draw Us a Picture

Set up your story by drawing us a picture. A quick phrase like "I could tell he had once been an athlete. Very muscular, except for the withered leg that no longer works."

Television news is always pressed to save time. But a well-told story can stretch those limits as part of a sound bite.

The Story is Convincing

Saying how you feel, and then telling your story reinforces your opinion and helps to get your point across.

You should have a library of transition phrases that smoothly take you to your story. Like:

- For instance ...

- Let me give you an example ...

- I wish you could have seen ...

- I came to that conclusion after I ...

- I didn't feel this way until I ...

Your Listening Face

During a webcam interview, we will also see you listening. Be aware of your facial expression while you're listening to the person on the other side of the conversation.

Your listening face needs to tell us that you're comfortable, self-confident, alert, glad to be here.

Without saying a word, you can also make a very strong statement by telegraphing that you agree - or vehemently disagree - with the person who is speaking at the other end of the connection.

Where Did That Idea Come From?

A frown or "what the hell" expression telegraphs that you think the person speaking is absolutely wrong. Or stupid.

A slight smile and nod puts your stamp of approval on whatever is being said at the other end of the conversation.

A laugh says your opponent's idea is truly crazy.

During Presidential debates, well-trained candidates have learned how to contradict and criticize their opponents without saying a word. In that format, the screen is often split so we can see both candidates.

As an opponent talks about a program or a position, we see the other candidate's face express disgust, dislike or astonishment with a smile, a nod, a frown, an eye roll.

The silent listening face can sometimes be more eloquent than the spoken word.

On-Camera Skills for Patients

For Telemedicine exams to succeed, the patients' ability to show and tell their symptoms is absolutely essential. In some cases, that skill can be even more critical for success than the equipment they're using.

Please excuse the repetition, because at this point, I'll need to repeat some of what I wrote in *On-camera Skills for Doctors and Nurses*. Some of the same basic stuff is necessary at both ends of a Telemedicine visit.

I assume medical professionals won't read this chapter, and patients won't read the professionals' chapter. So some of this material needs to be in both places.

It Seems So Simple

Telemedicine exams seem like such a simple idea. All you need to do as a patient is to sit in front of a camera and talk to your doctor or nurse.

WRONG.

Because something happens subconsciously when most of us first try to communicate on camera.

This is a learned skill.

When we are aware that we're being recorded, we become more cautious. We're not as spontaneous. We tend to talk louder, because the doctor or nurse is very far away.

We Don't Want to Be Embarrassed

We may not disclose some stuff, because it is embarrassing. Private. Even though we have almost total, legal protection that prevents others from knowing the details of our medical history, some patients still find it difficult to share everything with their doctor.

With Telemedicine, those cautious patients think:

All these intimate details about me will be recorded and just sitting there - I'm not sure where - but other people - I'm not sure who - will be able to see and hear what I said or did.

That's also true with old-fashioned medicine. Those details are sitting somewhere right now in a manila file folder. Photographs and X-rays, and written notes about what you told your physician.

But you trust your doctor to protect your privacy. The law says doctors can be sued, lose their license, perhaps prosecuted if your trust is violated.

Telemedicine & HIPPA Privacy

The same kinds of legal protection apply to what happens between you and your doctor through telemetry.

In 1996, Congress passed a new law that tied up a lot of loose ends to protect patients' medical privacy. The Health Insurance Portability and Accountability Act (HIPPA) applies nationwide. It is very strict.

If your doctor decides to use Telemedicine, the equipment and software have been rigorously built to HIPPA standards. The webcam the doctor supplies may look like the one you bought at Staples. But the software driving it will be MUCH more complicated and secure.

Learning with Simpler Gear

Meanwhile, your future visits with the doctor will be much more successful if you use an ordinary webcam for the learning process.

Be sure to read the chapter on *The Technical Stuff.* If you're using a built-in laptop webcam, I strongly recommend that you buy another webcam that will plug into your desktop computer, laptop or tablet. Plus a small tripod.

This will make it much easier to become familiar and proficient with the on-camera process.

Cheaper Than Doctor Visits

Total cost for the webcam and tripod will be less than $100. Much cheaper than two or three trips to the doctor's office.

Your doctor may even loan you this kind of equipment, then replace it with more secure gear after you've become comfortable with communicating this way.

Loss of Energy

One hurdle for Telemedicine is the subtle loss of energy that occurs when we watch someone on camera. I have interviewed thousands of people on camera.

And almost without exception, when I watched the replay, they were not as lively, not as engaging, not as effective as they were when I filmed the interview.

I know the camera is accurate. The camera has not distorted time or facial expression. It has not siphoned away sincerity or caring.

No, something happens in the *perception of the viewer*.

The Face Formula

In the chapter on *Creating Sound Bites*, you'll find my FACE formula. At the risk of being repetitive in that chapter, I'll tell you here that the E in that acronym stands for ENERGY.

You have probably had the experience of time slowing down in moments of great stress. It can happen as your car goes into a skid. Or you face a robber with a gun.

Tachypsychia

The technical term for it is tachypsychia. It is caused by:

- A dump of adrenalin in your bloodstream
- Total, focused attention

It is my theory that people are more boring on camera than they are in real life because the viewer has to focus more on what is being said onscreen that they would if the conversation was taking place in person.

Focusing on the replay triggers a tiny bit of tachypsychia.

So you have to invest more energy in what you say on camera, to correct the distortion.

The only way you can learn how much energy to invest is to watch yourself on camera.

And then practice enough so you know as you speak what you're projecting. That you will appear to be speaking in your normal tone of voice.

What the Doctor Needs to See & Hear

What the doctor needs to see and hear during your visit over the Internet will depend on the doctor's specialty, and your medical problem.

In virtually all cases, there will be portions of the visit where the doctor needs a sharp close-up of your face while you talk.

Your eyes and the way you speak can often disclose more than your words convey.

A psychiatrist or psychologist will probably want to see your entire body for most of the visit, because your body English transmits all sorts of information you may not be aware that you're sending.

Full-Body Shots

If the doctor wants to see your entire body, you'll need to be several feet away from the webcam. Most webcams have built-in microphones. If you're that far away, the sound will not be very good.

So you'll need a clip-on mic that plugs into your computer. There are lots of details on improving audio quality with an auxiliary mic, and where/what to buy in the chapters on *The Technical Stuff* and *Buying a Webcam*.

The Doctor as Director

From time to time, the doctor or nurse may ask you to change your position so they can better see something. Like:

- "Can you move a little closer to the webcam so I can see that place on your cheek a little better?

- "Yes, hold your arm right there for a moment. I want to take a picture of it."

- "Can you walk across the room now, and then come back. I need to see how that broken ankle is doing."

Equipment You Can Operate

In the chapter on *Telemedicine Tools*, There are some examples of tools already available to help in Telemedicine exams.

Doctor or Nurse Will Direct You

If you have been given this equipment, the doctor or nurse may say:

- "Now I need you to pick up that stethoscope and hold it against your chest so I hear your heart"

- "Just a little to the left now. Take in a deep breath and hold it." OR

- "You have a tool there that looks like a ballpoint pen with a wire on it. The other end has a little light. I'd like you to put the light inside your left nostril and hold it while I look around in there."

- "Now open your mouth wide, and point the light at the back of your throat as you say Aaaah."

The quality of video that these tools transmit is amazing. Just as good as if the doctor was holding the tool, instead of examining your sore throat a thousand miles away.

Learning to Say It Quickly

Telemedicine saves a huge amount of time. Particularly patient time in travel and the waiting room. But the time of the doctor or nurse is still limited.

So you need to think ahead about what you need to show and tell, once you're connected. It might be a good idea to have some notes handy near your webcam.

You need to learn how to summarize. I have a one-liner:

> The ultimate on-camera skill is learning how to tell the history of the human race in one sentence, without taking breath.

The Elevator Speech

This has also been called "the elevator speech." Tell me what I need to know in the time it takes the elevator to go from one floor to the next.

If doctors are interested in your summary, they'll ask a follow-up question. You'll be given more time to expand your thoughts.

What to Wear

Another wonderful asset for Telemedicine patients is that you don't have to get dressed. If you're spending long days recuperating in bed, wearing pajamas, that's fine.

You can comb your hair. Or not. Wear shoes or be barefoot.

Patients Intimidated

Many patients are intimidated when they're talking to a doctor or nurse in person. They forget to ask questions they planned before the exam. Once you get the hang of talking on camera, you'll probably find Telemedicine less intimidating.

It seems easier to ask embarrassing or off-the-wall questions online than it would be in person.

For most patients, it's easier in a Telemedicine exam than it is in person to plan ahead and collect stuff the doctor needs to see or hear.

With the camera in your cell phone, you can shoot pictures or video in a running medical diary, then show them to the doctor during the exam.

Revisiting the Exam

Another marvelous advantage of Telemedicine is the ability to record the visit with your doctor, and replay it later. There may be sections where you didn't quite understand what the doctor said.

Patients often don't want to admit they failed to grasp something. They don't want to look stupid.

With Telemedicine, you can go back privately and replay it until you DO understand.

The Technical Stuff

Telemedicine interviews/exams need these basic elements:

- Powerful computer
- High-speed internet connection
- High-quality webcam and the right framing
- High-quality microphone (which may be built-in)
- Simple auxiliary lighting
- Background that tells us something
- On-camera skills

Laptop Webcams

The webcams built into most laptops are not very good. Measuring the quality can get complicated, but here's a crude way to check:

Take a still picture with your laptop webcam. Then look at that picture in a photo editing or file managing program like File Explorer (Windows®) or Finder (the program that shows files in an Apple® computer). With your cursor over the file name, right click it.

A menu list will drop down. Left click PROPERTIES. You'll see a lot of stuff about the photo, including its dimensions in pixels. Pixels are the tiny dots that make up the photograph. The more pixels, the higher the image quality.

How to Measure Quality

Multiply the vertical pixels by the horizontal pixels. Most laptop webcams will shoot photos of about 2 MP (two million pixels).

By comparison, my separate USB webcam shoots 15 MP photos at 96 dpi (dots per inch). That's SEVEN TIMES more resolution that the average laptop webcam.

Be aware the dimensions of a still photograph shot by a webcam may not be the same as the video it shoots.

This is just a rough way to measure the quality of the webcam you're using, so you can compare it with the one you might buy.

The Computer

Your computer needs to be fairly new, and fast enough to process and transmit the video/audio signal your webcam produces. Here's how to find out what's inside the guts of your computer:

- If you have a Windows machine, go to CONTROL PANEL and click on SYSTEM.
- For an Apple computer, go to ABOUT THIS MAC.

Take Notes on Your System

Write down what you see there, because you'll need to know these things to make sure the webcam you shop for is compatible with your computer:

- Central Processing Unit (CPU) type and clock speed in GHz (gigahertz)
- Amount of RAM (random access memory) installed in GB (gigabytes)
- Operating System (OS) type

Windows comes in 32-bit and 64-bit versions.

Macs will show the Operating System (OS) as a name and number.

My desktop has an Intel® Quad Core™ CPU with a clock speed of 3.3 GHz. It's running Windows 10 (the 64-bit version) and has 16 GB of RAM. I built it from scratch. It is fast, and powerful.

Don't Be Intimidated

Don't be intimidated by the geek terms. You don't need to understand what they mean. Just be sure the webcam you buy will work with your computer.

If you want to use the best new webcam, you may need a newer, faster computer. One of the hurdles for webcam interviews is what we have come to expect from watching TV. Broadcast-quality cameras cost more than $50,000.

Those cameras produce VERY sharp video (unless the aging reporter or anchor tells the photographer to shoot slightly out of focus to blur the wrinkles). TV news cameras have near-perfect color balance, and true-to-life audio.

Webcams for Grandma & Lovers

Webcams and programs like Skype and Face Time were invented to let Grandma see and talk to the grandkids halfway across the country.

Or so young lovers could chat and see each other while they talk.

There was no need for anything fancy. Just a low price. Most Grandmas and young students have limited budgets.

More Sophisticated Now

As the industry began to realize webcam possibilities, more sophisticated webcams came to market. And as the quality increased, so did the price.

Then mass sales brought the prices down. My Logitech C920 (considered by most reviewers to be one of the best available) now costs about $70 online.

It has full HD capability, with 1080p resolution (1080 lines of pixels from top to bottom). I can choose HD screen proportions (9x16) or the old, standard proportions (2x3).

Search on the Internet

Begin your search for a webcam on the Internet. Using your favorite search engine, look for "best webcams." Read reviews published by technical magazines and blogs.

Once you've narrowed the list down to three or four webcams the reviewers recommend, go to websites that sell those models. Read reviews by owners who bought them there.

I'll recommend merchants in the chapter on _Buying Your Webcam_. Remember - you get what you pay for.

Don't Buy What You Don't Need

There are lots of webcam features out there you will never use. So don't buy what you don't need.

Here are the basic specifications I recommend:

- <u>USB connection</u> - This is the easiest way to connect the webcam to your computer. With one cable, you just plug it in. Most webcams have a built-in microphone designed to pick up your voice and suppress background noise.

- <u>Most webcams work fine with USB 2</u>. USB 3 (3rd generation) is about 40 times faster than USB 2. To take advantage of the faster speed, your computer must have plug-in sockets for USB 3. USB 3 is backwardly compatible. A USB 3 socket will have a blue insert. USB 2 sockets come in various colors.

- <u>Compatibility with your computer's OS</u> -This is why you need to know the basic operating system information for your computer. Some webcams will not work with some Apple or Linux® operating systems. Or an older Windows OS. Be sure to look for comments on OS compatibility in the user reviews at merchant websites.

- <u>Auto focus</u> - This keeps the camera focused sharply on whatever is at the center of the screen, no matter how far away it is from the camera. With some models, you can switch to manual focus and sharpen the picture by turning a ring on the lens or by moving a slider switch onscreen with your mouse. Cheap webcams have a fixed-focus lens that cannot be adjusted.

- <u>Ability to record at least 720p</u> (720 horizontal lines of onscreen pixels) - True HD (high definition) video is 1080p, but in many cases something in your data pipeline may prevent more than 720p from squeezing through. Your audio/video signal can be no faster or detailed than the slowest point in the data pipeline that transmits the webcam audio and video to the Internet.

- <u>Zoom lens</u> - This enables you to zoom in or out, and decide how much you want to capture in your webcam shot. Without it, the only way to control this is to move the webcam closer or farther away. Zooming is much better. It lets you sit farther away from the webcam but still fill the frame, so you won't be distorted, with an enlarged nose that appears to be pressed against the lens.

- Capable of taking still photos of at least 2 MP - With video editing software, you can pull a still photo from the video. With most webcams, you can take a still picture by pushing a button or clicking your mouse. Some webcams even give you a countdown on screen. In case you're taking your own picture, this gives you time to pose for the shot.

- Capable of producing at least 30 fps (frames per second) video - Some webcam video is jerky and out of synch because the webcam and computer are not capable of more than 15 fps. Movies and video are simply a series of still photos that flash very quickly and give us the illusion of movement. Thirty fps will give you smooth Internet video.

- A tripod socket - The webcam needs a tripod mounting socket. Many use a clamp that clips to the top of the monitor. A tripod socket will provide much more versatility for Telemedicine sessions. More about that later. You'll also need a small tripod that can sit on your desk in front of your monitor.

The Microphone

Many webcam interviews sound like the subject was in the shower and the microphone was out in the hallway. The closer to your mouth, the higher the quality of the sound it produces.

Most built-in webcam mics are designed to grab sound that's 16 to 20 inches away (about the distance from your monitor to your mouth) and muffle background noise.

Some even have two microphones to deliver more natural, stereo sound.

You can buy a top-of-the line webcam with a very good integrated microphone for less than it costs to buy a medium-priced webcam and a separate microphone.

It's also easier to install a webcam if the software and USB connection automatically merge audio and video.

Even so, for perfectionists who want the highest quality audio, a microphone closer to your mouth will do a better job. A small, clip-on mic, available online for about $30, is ideal.

Origin of the Sound

It will plug into the audio input jack of your computer. You'll have to set your sound system software so it knows where the audio is coming from.

They also make headsets like the ones sportscasters use, with a mic that comes around from one side and is positioned very close to your mouth. TV anchors and sportscasters often wear this kind of mic to minimize background noise. A clip-on is easier to use.

Try a webcam with a built-in microphone first. If you don't like what you hear, experiment and spend the money for a better solution.

The Internet Connection

The speed of your Internet connection is critical for great Telemedicine interviews. To be successful, you MUST have a fast connection.

Since the Internet was created, computer users have focused on download (receiving) speed. In the early years, ordinary computer users rarely uploaded (sent) data.

There was no Internet, e-mail or digital photography in the Dark Ages of computers. Nearly everyone now uploads photos and large documents to websites, or attached to e-mails. That makes upload speeds much more important.

Uploads 10 Times Slower

But most Internet service providers (ISPs) designed their systems around download speeds, not uploads. Their upload speeds are usually about one-tenth the download speeds. When you transmit video and audio with your webcam, you're uploading the data to the Internet, where it travels and is then downloaded to the computer at the other end of the conversation.

Telephone Dial-Up Won't Work

At the beginning of the computer age telephone lines let computers connect to one another. There are a few people in very isolated areas of the United States who still connect by telephone, but telephone modems can download data no faster than 56 kb/s (56,000 bits per second). More often, at less than 35 kb/s (35,000 bits per second).

That means upload speed of about 3.5 kb/s (3,500 bits per second). Not nearly fast enough for webcams. Even those who use a satellite system to connect from isolated areas may find their speed marginal for good webcam audio and video.

Don't worry about exactly what all this means. Everything that measures speed in the computer world is relative - compared to what?

Minimum Upload Speed

The best webcams today recommend an upload speed of at least 1 Mb/s (1 million bits per second). Even the slowest cable connections offer upload speeds several times faster. The cable company I use provides 1.5 Mb/s uploads for its slowest, cheapest Internet connection service.

I pay extra to get 100 Mb/s downloads and 10 Mb/s uploads.

However you connect to the Internet, you need to know your upload speed. Lots of websites can measure that for you, and it's free.

Use your search engine to look for "measure internet connection speed." Then go to some of the websites and follow directions.

Measuring Your Speed

The website I use most often to measure my upload and download speeds is www.speedtest.net. You should test your speed several times because speed of the same connection can vary from minute to minute.

Your Internet provider probably offers a website you can use to make sure they're providing the speed you're paying for. The higher the speed, the more they charge.

And the better your webcam signal will be.

Test at Several Websites

You might also want to check your speed at four or five different testing websites. The number of people surfing the Internet and the number of people using your ISP (Internet service provider) will cause speeds to vary at different times of day and different days of the week.

At most of the speed-testing websites, they're trying to sell you something that is supposed to make your computer faster. Don't be conned. You probably don't need it. But the tests are free.

LAN vs. Wi-Fi

Your fastest speed for both uploads and downloads will occur if your computer is connected by cable to your modem. This called a Local Area Network (LAN) connection. The plugs at both ends of a LAN cable look like a telephone plug, but a little larger.

If you connect wirelessly, the speed will usually be about half the LAN speed.

Good Lighting

The best of today's webcams can shoot in very dim light. But the better the lighting, the better the video will be. Bright lighting will provide much crisper video and a sense of three dimensions.

In the *Lighting and Background* chapter I'll show you how the placement of your lights is also critical to improve the quality of your webcam video.

Buying Your Webcam

I buy almost everything electronic online.

Online, you have the largest possible selection to choose from. Prices are lower than local stores. At some web merchants, you pay no sales tax. And they frequently offer free shipping.

Search for Reviews

If you decide to get a better webcam, the first step is to read a number of webcam reviews posted by technical magazines, blogs and forums. Search for "best webcams" or "webcam reviews."

Be aware that there may be a conflict of interest in some of these reviews. The magazine or online publication may carry advertising.

Consider the Advertising

The advertising can tilt reviews in favor of those brands. Sometimes manufacturers provide free products to be reviewed, and that can prejudice what's written about them.

You'll find that the best webcams are recommended by several reviewers. All of the reviewers can't be bought. When you have several highly rated models in mind, go to websites that sell those webcams.

The Manufacturer's Website

You may also want to go to the webcam manufacturer's website. There, you'll find the list price, and be able to better compare the features of different models they make.

A shortcut to find good prices and who sells them is to search for "price shopping services" or "price comparison services" with your favorite search engine.

How Price-Shopping Works

On the price-shopping website, you enter the brand and model number. They tell you where that item is for sale, and at what price. Some also give you customer ratings for the merchants they monitor.

Be aware, however, that price-shopping services don't cover every merchant. And the prices they post are often out of date.

I've learned to also use a search engine to look for the brand and model I want to buy. Sometimes that will turn up a merchant and a low price that's not listed by the price shopping services.

Rating Online Merchants

I rate online merchants by their:

- Low prices
- Return policies
- Customer service
- System for searching within their own website
- Collection of user reviews, and the ability to sort them (best to worst)
- Speed in shipping my order
- e-mailing me when my order is shipped, with a tracking number

Reviews by Customers

Most online merchants now collect reviews from ordinary people who have bought from them. I've come to depend on user reviews for critical information. Unless the merchant has posted phony customer reviews, they're fairly reliable.

I have more respect for reviews that include some really nasty comments while a high percentage of the reviewers praise the product. Reviews with no unsatisfied customers make me suspect the reviews have been censored.

Ordinary users tell you about software conflicts and lousy technical support if they had problems with installation. Professional reviewers are often too kind, not wanting to be cut off by a manufacturer if they're too critical.

Skill Level Tilts Reviews

Professional reviewers are also highly skilled in using computers. Something that seems easy to the pros may not be so simple for those who have less computer knowledge and experience.

The best of the user review systems also tell you how much technical expertise the reviewer claims.

Some of the terrible reviews often come from newbies (beginners) who simply didn't know how to install or use the equipment. Take those with a grain of salt. And understand that the best brands occasionally produce a defective item.

My Favorite Shopping Sites

My favorite websites for electronic gear are amazon.com and newegg.com. They have very good prices (especially if there's a sale or rebate) and a lot of free shipping.

You can set up an alert that will send you an e-mail if their price drops.

At almost all sites now, they remember you, once you've set up an account and ordered from them. That makes future purchases very easy.

Always Use a Credit Card

I always use a credit card for online purchases. If something goes wrong between you and the merchant, most credit card companies will stop payment until you're satisfied.

If your credit card company is not willing to be your advocate, you need to cancel that card and get another.

Many people are concerned about the security of using a credit card online. I'm much more concerned about a waiter in a restaurant copying my credit card number, then using it to increase the tip, or buy something else with the card. I've had that happen.

Credit Card Security

Most credit card companies protect their card holders from fraud. They have very good security systems. In a city away from home, I bought some clothing at two different stores one morning. When I was checking out at a third store, my cell phone rang.

The call was from American Express®, checking to make sure my card had not been stolen.

More recently, I was at home when I paid $350 online to a company in London. American Express called in less than a minute to ask if the charge was legitimate. I was amazed that their system had flagged the purchase and reacted so swiftly.

Extended Warranties

Some credit cards will double the manufacturer's warranty (up to an extra year) for anything you buy with them.

I've collected on the extended warranty feature at least a half-dozen times. But beware - if you buy the merchant's extended warranty, the credit card warranty extension will usually no longer apply.

Some merchants and some credit card companies have a price-match policy. If something you buy goes on sale within a month or so, they'll refund the difference between that and what you paid.

Unpack it Carefully

When you buy your webcam, unpack it very carefully and save EVERYTHING that came with it. If it's defective, or incompatible with your computer, you won't be able to return it unless everything that came with it goes back to the merchant.

Use a Large Screen

For Telemedicine, always use the largest screen you have. A cell phone screen is much too small to handle the detail that's needed. Tablets are only a little better.

The monitor for my desktop is a 27-incher. The computer in my entertainment system connects to a TV set (shown on the front cover of this book) that measures 65 inches diagonally.

The nurse photographed holding her stethoscope to the screen was shot tongue-in-cheek, but that size screen would be very helpful to a doctor or nurse examining a patient by Skype.

Installing Your Webcam

First, read the directions that came with your webcam. ALL OF THEM. To save money, most electronics manufacturers no longer print long directions. The extensive instructions are either online or on the CD that comes with the product.

Don't Use the Disk Until ...

But DON'T use the enclosed CD to install the webcam until you've checked the manufacturer's website. This technology is evolving so rapidly, that enclosed disk is probably out of date.

Go to the manufacturer's website. Click on SUPPORT or DOWNLOADS. Find the file that installs your webcam on your type of operating system.

It will show a version number and a date. Compare that to the version printed on the CD. If they're the same, it's easier to use the disk. If the website version is newer, download the file.

Updates Avoid Problems

Software is constantly updated to fix bugs. When enough buyers call technical support about a problem with their hardware of software, the company finds what it will take to solve the problem, and releases a new version.

You can save yourself a lot of time and trouble if you have the latest version. A small program that runs a piece of computer hardware like a printer or a webcam is called a "driver."

Don't Lose the Download

You need to know where the file is after the download is finished. Some people download to their desktop. But if you do very much downloading, your desktop will become terribly cluttered.

Your browser may save all your downloads and make them easy to access.

I've set up my browser (Mozilla Firefox) so that all downloads go into a folder I created - C:\Downloads.

Once a software driver is in the Downloads folder, I move it to another folder:

C:\Software Updates\Manufacturer's Name. I do it that way because I sometimes need to install the same update on several computers.

Or, if a program becomes corrupted, I can re-install it without having to download it again. When the next update is issued, I put it in that folder and delete the older file.

Reduce the Chance of a Glitch

Once you have the driver downloaded and you know where it is, shut down all programs that are running. Some programs will tell you to do this; others won't.

Having all programs turned off will reduce the chance of a glitch in the installation.

Put your cursor on the file name and double-click it. That will start the installation of the program. Follow the on-screen directions.

Wait to Plug In Your Webcam

Don't plug in your webcam until the installation software tells you to. Most webcams are designed to sit on top of your monitor. Put it there for the install.

With the installation finished, and the webcam plugged in, launch the program (if it's not already running). You should see yourself on screen, sitting in front of your monitor.

A star is born.

Go Through the Setup Process

The first time you turn on the webcam, most installation software will take you through a setup routine to adjust the video and audio settings. You'll have to tell the computer if you're using a microphone that's not integrated in the camera. And where it's plugged in.

Only one program can use the webcam at a time. If another program has automatically started as a result of your plugging in the webcam, you'll have to close it to adjust the initial settings for the webcam.

Most of the manufacturers' programs give you a chance to make a test video and then play it back.

Solving Sound Problems

If there's no sound on the playback, you probably haven't designated the right mic and/or audio input jack.

Be aware that the dictionary now includes two ways to spell the shortcut name for a microphone. It was originally mike. A second, acceptible way to spell it is now MIC.

Installing Skype

Skype is the leading program that connects one webcam user to another for a video call. You'll need to become a Skype member and download their software to use the service. It's free. Most TV news operations use Skype.

With your Internet browser, go to http://www.skype.com. On their website, you may have to do a little searching to find the button that downloads the program for your operating system. Skype is now owned by Microsoft.

Video Calls are Free

Video calls between Skype members are free, no matter where they are, anywhere in the world. The Skype website is cluttered with offers for you to subscribe to their paid calling service.

Don't be confused by those ads.

Don't Pay for Regular Phone Calls

The calling service they're trying to sell you uses Skype to make a regular telephone call. The call they charge for is just a regular telephone call, to a regular telephone number, which uses your computer's speakers and microphone.

It's really just another form of speaker phone.

Skype calls the phone number and if someone answers, plugs the connection into your account at Skype.

You pay by the minute. It's probably cheaper than using your telephone for an international call, but not free.

A Skype video call is free, and much better, in my opinion.

Searching for Skype Members

Once you've signed up, you can log in and search for other Skype members by name and location, or by e-mail address. When you find a person you might want to call, put them in your Skype contact list.

With the list showing and your webcam plugged in, clicking on the contact's name turns on your webcam and makes the call.

Placing or Answering a Call

If they're at their computer, with Skype running in the background, you'll connect almost instantly. They can answer the call with a mouse click.

Their face will fill your screen. The image your webcam is transmitting will be in a small box at the corner of your screen. That's so you can see the video you're sending, and adjust where the camera is pointing, if necessary.

You Can Choose Standby

If they don't have Skype running in the background, or choose not to answer, you'll get a message that says there was no answer.

If you want to be constantly available for others to call you on Skype, you should choose the option of launching Skype each time you turn on your computer.

If you've made all the right settings, you and the person on your screen can carry on a conversation that's sorta like being in the same room with each other.

For as long as you like. Absolutely free. This is how troops stationed overseas stay in touch with their families. Truly astounding technology.

Check Skype's Drain

When it's running in the background, Skype uses three percent of my computer's available RAM.

If you want to check how many resources it's using on your Windows computer when Skype is minimized, hold down the CTRL and ALT keys, then touch DELETE.

The Task Manager window will pop up. Click the PRO-CESSES tab. It will show how hard your CPU is working, and how much RAM is being used. With the Task Manager window still in view, close Skype and note how that affects both CPU and RAM resources.

Checking Resources On an Apple

On an Apple computer, go to APPLICATIONS, then UTILI-TIES, then ACTIVITY MONITOR to see how your webcam program is affecting RAM and CPU resources.

There are also a number of small programs (sometimes called "widgets") for both Windows and Apple machines that will give you more detailed information on how a program is using your system's resources. Use a search engine to find these widgets and download them.

Other Video Calling Programs

There are other video calling programs like Skype. Apple's version is Face Time. But because Skype was the pioneer in this field, it has the most users. So most of your interviews will probably use Skype. Instead of connecting through a telephone line, you're using the Internet as the connection route.

After you've had some experience with Skype, you might want to try other programs. Some may work better with your equipment.

No matter which system you use, both ends of the conversation must be using the same program.

Webcam Placement

If your webcam is perched on top of your desktop monitor, it's probably looking down its nose at you. A computer in your lap with a built-in webcam will usually be looking up your nostrils.

There are better ways to place your webcam.

We Expect Eye Contact

In normal conversations, we expect to have eye contact with the other person. In this culture, this is REALLY, REALLY important.

That's one reason webcam interviews often seem strange. You're making eye contact with the image of the person on your monitor screen, but it appears to them that you're looking up or down, depending on where the webcam is sitting.

A Suspicious Look

If you're not making eye contact, we suspect you're not being honest. More about that in the *On-Camera Skills* chapters.

If the conversation takes place at a party and the other person has a wandering eye, we think they're searching for someone else who's more attractive or less boring.

If you're looking down at my chest (as it appears, if the webcam is too high) I wonder if I spilled something on my shirt. A woman wonders if you're captivated by her cleavage.

Eye Contact Illusion

If you're looking into the lens, at the other end of the line it appears that you're making direct eye contact.

So if the webcam is sitting on top of your monitor, you may need to change the height of the monitor or your chair. But that may not completely solve the eye contact issue.

A Better Idea

A better idea - buy a small tripod and put the webcam in front of the monitor, rather on top of it.

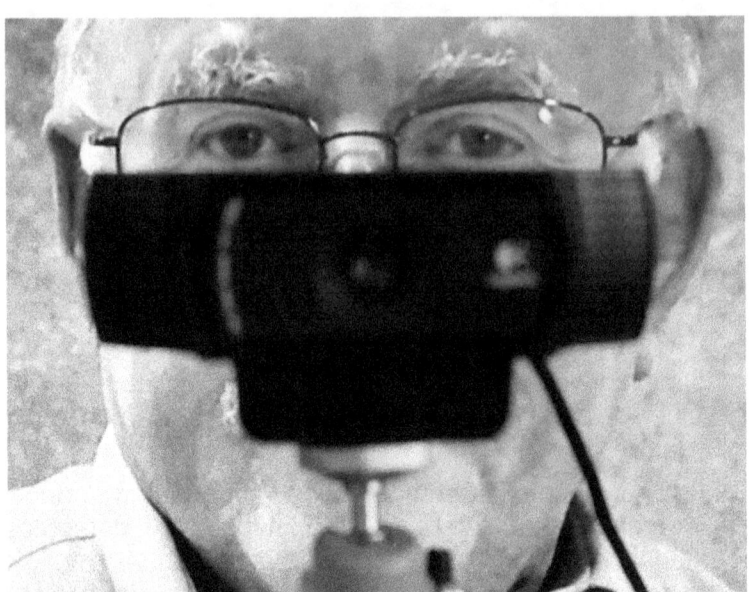

Setting Tripod Height

The easiest way I've found to deal with the eye contact issue is to adjust the tripod height so the lens of the webcam is just under the eyes of the person onscreen that you're talking to (above).

If your gaze skims across the top of the webcam as you look into the other person's eyes, it appears at their end that you're making direct eye contact.

The webcam and tripod will block some of their face, if they're very close to their camera, as in this shot. They'll probably be farther away in most Telemedicine conversations.

If you're the doctor or nurse, the eye contract illusion can be very important to build patient confidence at the beginning of the session. And this camera placement puts the built-in mic a lot closer to you for better audio quality.

Shifting for the Exam

During the actual exam, you will probably ask the patient to shift or move their webcam to give you a better look. For that part of the session, eye contact is not a critical factor.

If you're too close to the camera, there may be some unusual - sometimes comical - distortion of your face. Your nose can grow and appear to be pressed against the lens.

Here's where a zoom lens makes a higher-quality camera a bargain. You can sit farther away to avoid the close-up distortion, and zoom in so you still fill the camera frame.

The Distance Dilemma

Being farther away can seriously degrade the sound of your voice. Even with the special design of built-in webcam mics.

Test it. If your voice doesn't sound right, try a mic that's closer to your mouth. Some very good $10 mics can sit on the edge of the desk, in front of your keyboard.

The best solution is a clip-on mic. The kind you see TV anchor people wearing. It will always be close to your mouth, no matter where the camera sits.

Clip-ons are available now for about $30, and the quality of the sound they produce at that price point is surprisingly good.

Mic and Speaker Placement

Also be aware that the placement of the mic, in relation to your speakers, can cause audio feedback. An ear-splitting screech or squeal.

This is especially true if your speakers and the webcam are both built into the monitor.

If you use external speakers, put them at the back edge of your desk. Feedback will be much less likely there.

Don't forget that if you're in your home, a crying baby, a barking dog, or a ringing telephone can be a major distraction during a webcam interview.

If you think about it ahead of time, the barking dog and the ringing phone can be avoided. Babies are more difficult.

Lock the Door

So lock the door.

In March, 2017, Robert E. Kelly, a professor of political science in South Korea, was being interviewed by the BBC via webcam, discussing the impeachment of the South Korean President.

Kelly was unaware when his daughter, Marion, swung open the door behind him and pranced into the room. She was having a good time, celebrating after a birthday party.

Hi, Dad - Surprise!

Then Kelly's younger child, James, rolled into the room in a bouncer. Dad still did not know he had visitors. (below)

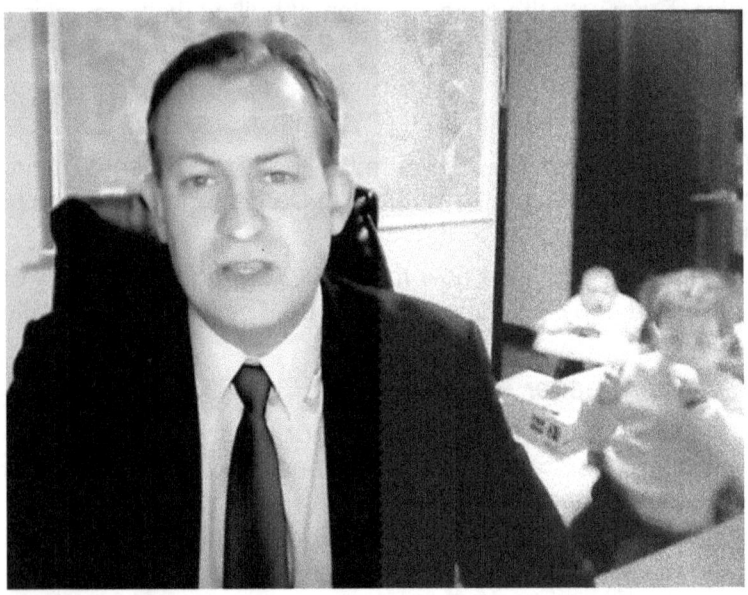

Moments after this shot was taken, Kelly discovered he was not alone. He smiled, a little embarrassed, and apologized to the BBC correspondent.

Then Kelly's frantic wife shot into the room, almost crawling, as she tried to stay out of the shot and drag the kids out the door.

Two days later, CBS reported the event had already been seen by 86 million viewers on YouTube.

It was wonderful entertainment.

Lighting & Background

Most ceiling lights put your eyes in deep shadow. It's important that we see your eyes. Television stations spend tens of thousands of dollars on experts who regularly fine-tune the lighting in their studios.

Lighting makes a huge difference in how we perceive people on camera.

Window Disadvantages

If your desk is near a window, placing the monitor so the window is behind it will use the light coming through the window to light your face. But only during daylight hours.

And you probably don't want to keep your monitor in that position all the time. Strong backlight makes it very hard to see what's on a computer monitor.

Auxiliary Lights

A better solution is one or two auxiliary lights that you'll use only for webcam interviews. Portrait photographers consider light from several directions absolutely essential if the photo is going to flatter their subjects.

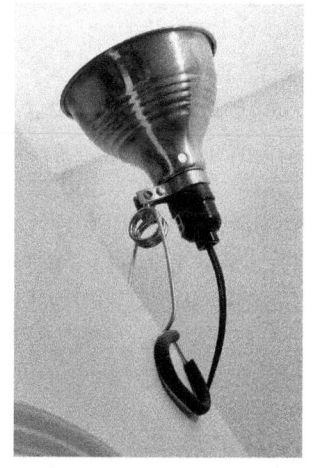

Almost any lights will work. They don't have to be very bright or costly. Webcams are designed to work with normal indoor lighting.

Utility lights they sell at hardware stores (right) are a great solution. They're about $10 each. They have a reflector, a push-button switch, and they come with a spring-loaded clamp that makes them easy to position.

LED bulbs are ideal for this kind of fixture. They won't get hot, and they come in several colors, to match the existing lighting in the room.

White Balance

However you light the webcam interview, something photographers call "white balance" is critical. Daylight is much bluer than incandescent lights. Fluorescent lights are closer to daylight, but come in several varieties.

If you use LED bulbs for auxiliary lighting, they also come in a variety of colors. If the other lights in the room are standard incandescents, use a warm white LED.

Try not to mix different colors of light in the same room. If the existing lights are fluorescents, use an LED that matches. Daylight LEDs will probably do it, but different brands labeled "daylight" vary greatly. You'll have to experiment.

The White Paper Test

To help your webcam transmit more accurate color, hold a white sheet of paper near the webcam so the paper fills the entire screen.

Then move the paper away. This can help the webcam adjust so the color is more natural. This will work with some webcams, not with others.

Better webcams will have a setup function to let you tweak the color balance, just as you do with a TV set. When your lights are in place, fine-tune the camera.

Another Tuning Test

Another way to test your color balance is to put a white sheet of paper under your chin, so you can see both your face and the paper.

This will sometimes help a webcam with automatic white balancing. Does the paper appear to be truly white? What did it do to your skin color when you added it to the shot?

Make a test recording and then hold the paper next to the monitor so you can see if what's on screen is the same white you recorded. If not, do some more tuning.

Beware the tiny LED indicator in some webcams that tell you the camera is turned on. They're usually red or blue, and may be bright enough to make your face that same shade of red or blue. If it changes the color balance, put a piece of opaque tape over the LED indicator.

Bounce Lighting

Here are some other ideas on how to light your set –

If your ceiling is white, point a light at a spot on the ceiling above where you'll be sitting, just a little in front of directly overhead. This is called "bounce lighting."

Try moving the light higher and lower to see how that affects what you see on camera. The soft, diffused light bounced off the ceiling will usually look like ordinary room lighting.

Raccoon Eyes

But because the bounced light is coming from directly over-head, it can create shadows under your eyes. Photographers call it "raccoon eyes."

To fix that, bounce a second light off the wall behind the webcam, a little to one side. IF the wall is white.

If it's not, tape some white paper or poster board to the wall, and place the light close to it. This will fill in the shadows from the overhead light, and put a glint in your eyes.

A Very Small Fill Light

A small desktop light can also provide the fill that removes the shadows under your eyes. Sometimes a bulb no brighter than a flashlight will do the trick.

To light like a pro, use a third light in a far corner of the room behind you, very high, and out of camera range. It should not be very bright.

This will give a live, three-dimensional look to the shot. If possible, adjust the brightness of the lights so you're well-lit and the background is darker.

Brighter Looks Sharper

The brightness of your lighting will affect the F-stop or aper-ture of the camera. Aperture is a photographic measurement of the size of the hole that lets light into the camera. If the light is bright, the aperture gets smaller, just like the iris in the human eye.

At this smaller aperture, the "depth of field" is larger. Depth of field is the distance at which objects in the video appear to be sharply in focus. With very bright lighting and a very small aperture, *everything* in the entire room will be in sharp focus.

If the lighting is dim, the aperture gets bigger. The depth of field decreases. Everything on-screen may seem less sharp.

Internet Lighting Tutorials

For more lighting ideas, search "portrait lighting" on the Internet. At many websites, the pros show the techniques they use to make people more attractive than they are in real life.

With a webcam, you get to see what you look and sound like. Make some test recordings and play them back. Adjust the lights until you're happy with them.

Dimmers Create Orange Light

If you use a dimmer on a light, be aware that the light will become more orange as the brightness decreases. Instead of a dimmer, try bulbs of different wattages.

Some of the light should be stronger, some more subtle. Try a white umbrella or poster board to bounce light from different directions.

Be careful if you're using incandescent or halogen lights. They can quickly get hot enough to set fabric or paper on fire. LED lights produce no heat. Their cool temperatures and the variety of color choices make them ideal for webcam auxiliary lighting.

The Background

This can be a difficult decision in setting up your webcam for interviews from your home or office. Should the background be plain or busy?

Lawyers and judges like to have a bookcase full of books behind them. It suggests they've read all of them, and they are, therefore, true experts.

In the early days of TV news, the wall behind the anchor desk was blank, or looked like a window to the city where the broadcast originated.

More recently, the consultants have added busy back-grounds. I'm not sure why. During some newscasts, we see a working newsroom behind TV anchors, filled with staff at keyboards and computer screens.

The newsroom in the background suggests that the anchor is the leader of a dedicated, hard-working team that is diligently gathering and producing stories for you.

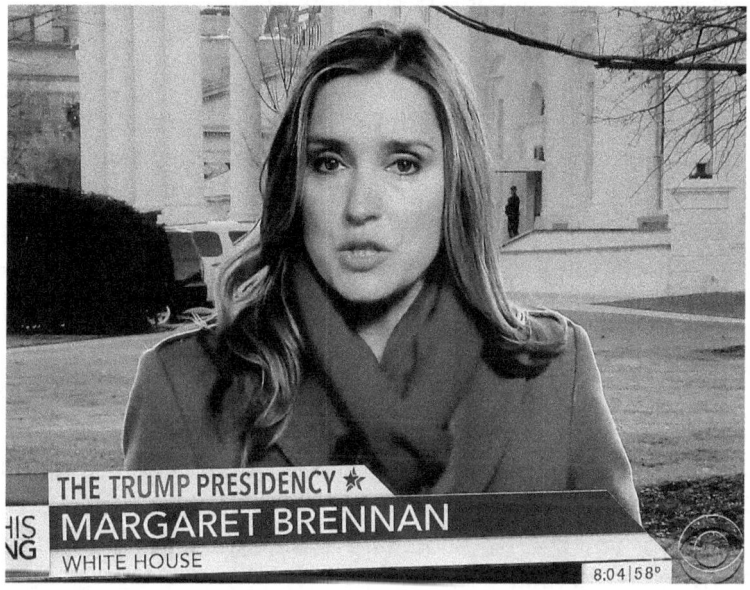

THE TRUMP PRESIDENCY ★
MARGARET BRENNAN
WHITE HOUSE
8:04 | 58°

White House Standups

Did you ever wonder why network TV correspondents do their standups (above) in front of the White House? The networks have studios a few blocks away that are air conditioned, sound-proof, and well-lit.

TV Studios Would Be Easier

The studios would be a much better place for high-quality video. During the winter, it gets dark in Washington before the nightly network news at 6:30 pm.

The shot on the White House lawn requires lighting. Sometimes, it's raining. Or snowing. It can be noisy.

There are often people walking in the background.

Subliminal Messages

They do their standups there because having the White House in the background delivers a subliminal message.

It makes the viewer believe the correspondents have been inside the White House all day, and now they're going to tell us exactly what's going on in there.

The right background lends authority to what you say.

Medical Messages

For Telemedicine, if you're a doctor or nurse, find a spot for your webcam that clearly shows you are in a doctor's office or medical facility. With maybe some lab equipment in the background.

If you're in pediatrics, let us see something that indicates children are often in your office. If you're in orthopedics, exercise equipment might provide a subliminal message.

Make It Simple

If the background can't help with the impression you'd like to give, make it as plain as possible. Like a blank wall.

The surface on the walls of cubicles in large offices are often covered with a carpet-like material that is ideal.

Whatever you choose should have a matte surface. Nothing shiny to create reflections.

A Fabric Backdrop

A lightweight blanket can make an easy, inexpensive backdrop. They come in all sorts of colors. Two yards of terry-cloth material from a fabric store will also work.

A twin-sized sheet is about the right size, but it's difficult to use because the wrinkles will show.

A dark color will usually work best. More about color in a moment. Other ideas to fill the space behind you in the webcam shot:

- An inflatable mattress sitting on end and covered by fabric can be propped against a chair to make an easy, portable backdrop.

- If one side of the mattress is flocked, and the color is right, you might even be able to use that side of the mattress without the fabric.

- If you work in a cubicle, the fabric can be draped over the wall behind you.

- If your desk is in the right place, the fabric can be clipped to the bracket that holds vertical blinds behind you. Blinds or drapes can also be the plain backdrop.

An Inexpensive Frame

It's easy to make an inexpensive frame with PVC pipe that will hold your fabric. It can be quickly assembled and taken apart. See how to make one in *Build a Backdrop Frame*.

The farther away the plain backdrop, the better - for shadows, as well as camera focus. In an ideal setup, you'll be in sharp focus and the backdrop will be fuzzy.

Most webcams are completely automatic, in terms of exposure. You don't have the ability to change the camera aperture and depth of field.

Lighting/Depth of Field Conflict

So with an automatic camera, you may have a conflict between good lighting and depth of field. The brighter the light, the smaller the aperture.

The smaller the aperture, the greater the depth of field. Everything behind you may be in very sharp focus.

If we're distracted by something in the background, you didn't do a very good job in your setup. Nothing should detract from you and your message.

Color and Automatic Exposure

With automatic exposure, the camera measures the lightness and darkness of everything in the entire shot and comes up with an average that sets the aperture.

If you have a white wall or fabric as the backdrop, the camera reacts the way your eye would - Wow! It's bright in here! - and the aperture stops down.

The camera shot makes it look like you've turned down the lights in the room. The smaller aperture changes depth of field. Everything in the room will be sharply in focus.

A dark background has the opposite effect. The camera thinks - Wow! It's dark in here! - and the aperture opens up. Your face can look washed out, like you're caught in a powerful spotlight, while everything else looks normal. The larger aperture will make the background less sharp.

Tailored Exposure

So the goal is to set up a background that makes the webcam auto exposure just right for your complexion.

A test question - If you have very dark skin, should the background be light or dark? The answer is counter-intuitive.

The correct answer: Dark. The webcam's measure of light and darkness in the entire frame will trigger a wider aperture in the webcam, and light your face better than it would with a lighter background.

With a light background, the details of your face can be almost invisible.

If you're extremely pale, a light background can make it look like you have a healthy tan.

Testing to Make it Right

There is no magic formula. The only way to find out what's right for you is to test different shades of light and dark until you find the right one.

Color itself is not that important for exposure. It is *lightness* and *darkness* that make the difference.

There's more about color and what to wear in the *On-Camera Skills* chapters.

Telemedicine Resources

The Internet is an incredibly rich resource if you want to know more about Telemedicine. The technology is expanding so rapidly, this book, in either printed or electronic form, was out of date an hour after it was last revised.

You'll find extensive websites offering or explaining Telemedicine from doctors, medical schools, hospitals, insurance companies, equipment, consulting and software firms.

To give you some idea of what's out there, a Google search for "Telemedicine" in mid-2017 returned 5,940,000 hits. Here are some short excerpts from the home pages of a few Telemedicine websites. They will, hopefully, get you started and encourage you to dig deeper:

The American Telemedicine Assn.

http://www.americantelemed.org/home

*ATA is a non-profit association based in Washington DC with a membership network of more than 10,000 industry leaders and healthcare professionals. We are a leading telehealth association helping to transform healthcare by improving the **quality**, **equity** and **affordability** of healthcare throughout the world.*

Today, the use of telemedicine has spread rapidly and is now becoming integrated into the ongoing operations of hospitals, specialty departments, home health agencies, private physician offices as well as consumer's homes and workplaces. It's no wonder why this has become a multibillion-dollar industry and why nearly every major hospital and healthcare system leverages it to transform and to reinvent healthcare.

*As the largest telehealth-focused organization, we offer the largest, international telehealth conference in the industry. We also feature the world's busiest web portal, the top eNewsletter, and the most-watched, monthly video series. ATA is also widely recognized for the unique, high quality **Advocacy-Education-Network** opportunities we offer.*

eVisit, LLC

https://evisit.com/what-is-telemedicine/

Telemedicine is a relatively new concept, and in the world of internet, it develops with lightning speed. This article is for those who want to understand all intricacies of this highly dynamic and fascinating field.

Table of Contents:

U.S Health and Human Services - HIPAA

https://www.hhs.gov/hipaa/for-individuals/guidance-materials-for-consumers/index.html

Most of us believe that our medical and other health information is private and should be protected, and we want to

know who has this information. The Privacy Rule, a Federal law, gives you rights over your health information and sets rules and limits on who can look at and receive your health information. The Privacy Rule applies to all forms of individuals' protected health information, whether electronic, written, or oral. The Security Rule is a Federal law that requires security for health information in electronic form.

Federal Communications Commission

https://www.fcc.gov/general/telehealth-telemedicine-and-telecare-whats-what

When thinking about healthcare, most of us conjure up images of office visits or trips to the ER. Whether it's for a routine check-up, lab tests, an outpatient procedure or major surgery, the norm is for patients and caregivers to leave their homes (often sitting in traffic or rushing from work) to meet their doctor at a healthcare facility of some kind. But things are changing.

Based on advances in information and communications technologies, medical professionals as well as other "health and care" providers can now offer increasingly robust, remote (from their location to another), interactive (two-way) services to consumers, patients and caregivers.

The terms used to describe these broadband-enabled interactions include telehealth, telemedicine and telecare. "Telehealth" evolved from the word "telemedicine." "Telecare" is a similar term that you generally hear in Europe. All three of these words are often - but not always - used interchangeably. They can also have different meanings depending on who you ask. And that's precisely why you should ask your doctor, your insurance provider, your nurse, anyone who's part of your health and care universe ...

U.S. Dept. HHS August, 2016 Report to Congress

https://aspe.hhs.gov/system/files/pdf/206751/TelemedicineE-HealthReport.pdf

The availability of telehealth is of particular interest for patients who live in areas that are inadequately served. Access to certain medical specialties, such as oncologists, is limited

in rural areas. Currently, 59 million Americans reside in Health Professional Shortage Areas (HPSAs), rural and urban areas with shortages of primary care providers. Of special concern are rural individuals who have higher mortality rates; a greater chance of being unnecessarily hospitalized; and have one-third as many specialists per capita as do persons living in cities.

Telehealth appears to hold particular promise for chronic disease management. Almost 50 percent of all adults in the United States have at least one chronic illness. Chronic disease accounts for approximately 75 percent of all health care expenditures and contributes to about 70 percent of all deaths in this country. Many persons with chronic conditions are elderly, and therefore have mobility limitations. Moreover, people with multiple chronic conditions typically require frequent visits to clinicians. Ensuring ready access to care for such individuals may help avert costly emergency room visits or hospital stays. However, aside from care for mental health, the majority of telehealth provided for chronic conditions to date has been limited to asynchronous monitoring.

AMA Code of Medical Ethics Chapter 1.2.12

https://www.ama-assn.org/delivering-care/ama-code-medical-ethics (adopted in June, 2016)

Physicians who provide clinical services through telehealth/telemedicine must uphold the standards of professionalism expected in in-person interactions, follow appropriate ethical guidelines of relevant specialty societies and adhere to applicable law governing the practice of telemedicine. In the context of telehealth/telemedicine they further should:

Be proficient in the use of the relevant technologies and comfortable interacting with patients and/or surrogates electronically.

Recognize the limitations of the relevant technologies and take appropriate steps to overcome those limitations. Physicians must ensure that they have the information they need to make well-grounded clinical recommendations when they cannot personally conduct a physical examination.

Telemedicine Tools

If you like gadgets, you'll go absolutely crazy when you see the hundreds of clever tools now available for Telemedicine exams.

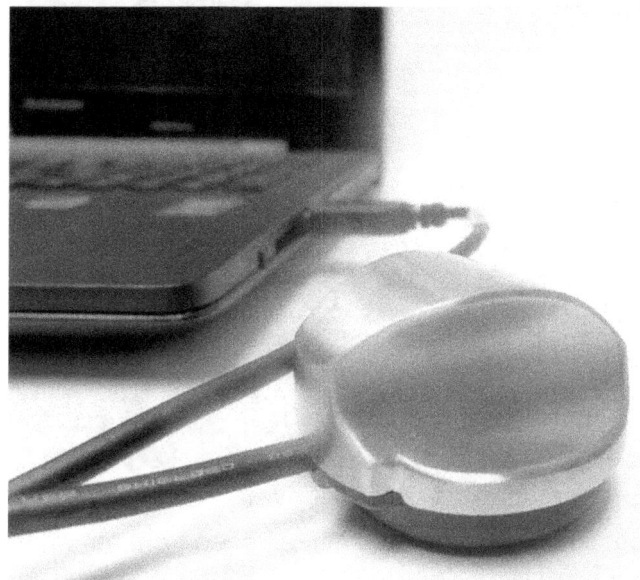

Like this stethoscope. The patient, in front of a Skype camera, plugs the stethoscope into a computer USB port.

The doctor or nurse (who's watching the patient do all this by webcam) tells the patient where to place the stethoscope.

Long-Distance Heartbeats

At the other end of the connection, the doctor or nurse says, "Now take a deep breath and hold it." They can hear exactly what they would hear if they were pressing the sensor against the patient's chest themselves.

Even better - with this device, they can turn up the volume or filter the signal to hear faint sounds that might not be audible at all with an old-fashioned stethoscope.

"OK, now breathe normally," the doctor says.

Amazing.

Here's another one. You know the gadget doctors have with a tiny light on the end? The one they use to look up your nose, or inside your ear?

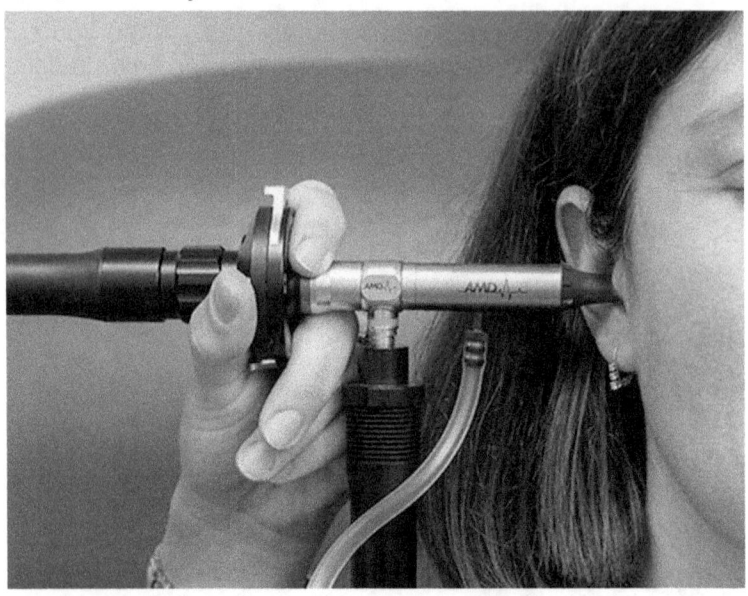

Here's the Telemedicine version (above).

And the patient's ear canal (below), as seen from anywhere on the planet.

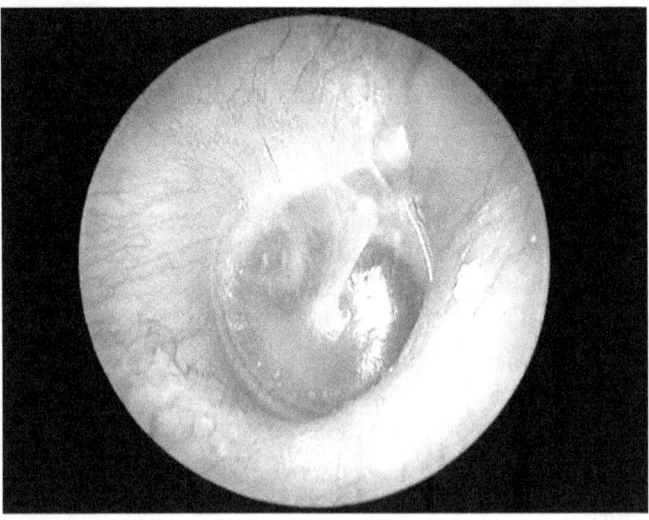

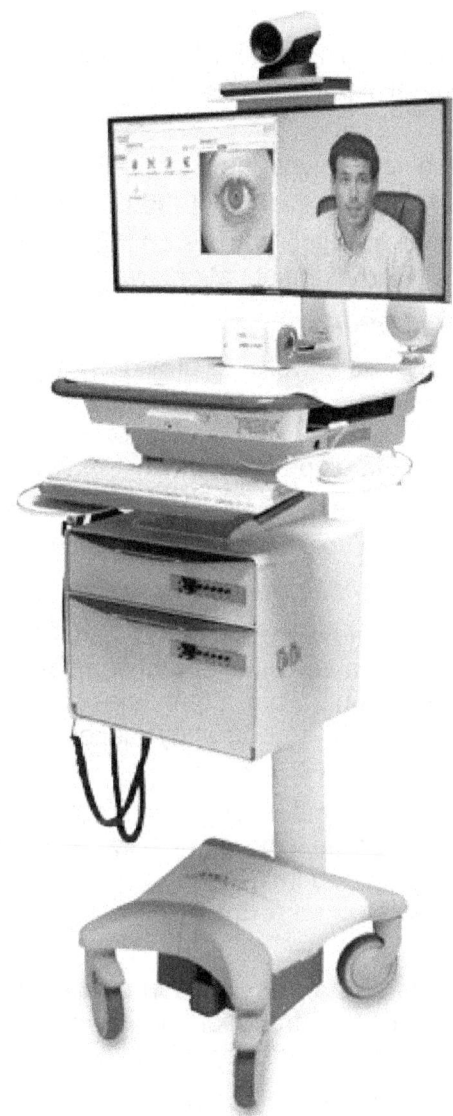

Peanuts, Popcorn, Crackerjacks

This rolling Telemedicine cart can move from one bed to another in a hospital or nursing home, so doctors far away, from a variety of specialties, can visit with the patients, check their vital signs, and see how they're doing.

In-Person Backup

Many doctors practicing Telemedicine prefer that a nurse or technician be with the patient when the doctor is connected by webcam.

The nurse or technician gives the exam a human touch, and can expand what the doctor sees through telemetry.

But as you can see from the devices on the previous pages, many can be operated by most patients without help.

AMD Global Telemedicine

The devices shown here were all provided by AMD Global Telemedicine in Chelmsford, Massachusetts. I discussed them with Dan McCafferty, AMD's vice president in charge of global sales and development.

He was demonstrating the equipment at the American Telemedicine Association's 2017 national convention.

Advanced Medicine in Primitive Places

"We're bringing very advanced medical care" he said, "To small, isolated communities all over the world where there is no doctor, no hospital, no clinic. Sometimes they have just a nurse-practitioner. And the geography makes it virtually impossible for a patient to see a doctor.

"Sometimes, it's an island nation, with scores of islands scattered in all directions. There's just no way for the few doctors they have to reach a patient who urgently needs care when he's isolated on a dot of land hundreds of miles away."

He said AMD does a lot of business in countries where the mountains are so rugged, transportation from rural areas to cities with medical facilities is impossible.

Telemedicine has no geographic limits.

Market research firms are predicting the U.S. telehealth market will reach $1.9 billion in 2018, and will continue growing in the near future at a rate of 56 percent ($1 billion) every year.

Build a Backdrop Frame

I've found two ways to create a plain backdrop for webcam interviews. Each is a square frame made with PVC pipe and fittings. You can hang fabric on it to hide the junk behind you in the room. They're easy to assemble and take apart. The pieces can easily be stored.

Back of Your Chair

The first is 48 inches square, and will fit over the back of your chair. It's a little bulky to store when it's not in use, but is really simple to use. Just slide it over the chair back and it's ready to go. This kind of backdrop is available online (below) for about $50.

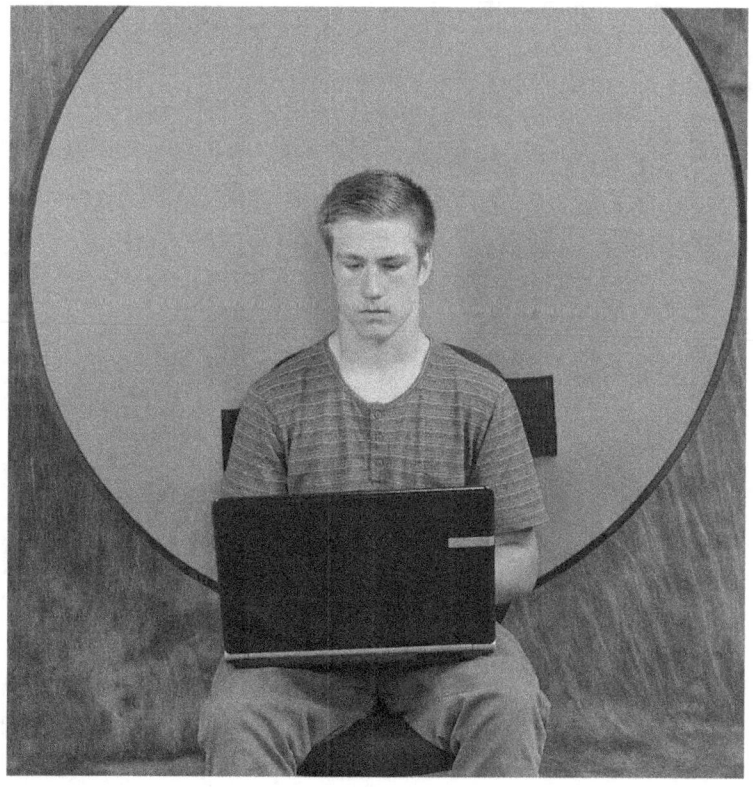

Ready-Made

The disadvantage of this type backdrop is how close it is to you. Both your face and the backdrop will be in sharp focus. More about that later in this chapter, and in the *Lighting and Background* chapter.

Building Your Own

Building our own with PVC pipe and fittings will cost about $10, two hours of time, and some measuring skills. Use ¾-inch PVC Schedule 40 pipe and fittings.

<u>FIRST STEP</u> - The first step is to make an assembly that will fit over the back of the chair you'll be using for webcam interviews.

The measurements will depend entirely on both the thickness and the width of the chair back. Making this module (let's call it the CHAIR MOUNT) will take some trial and error.

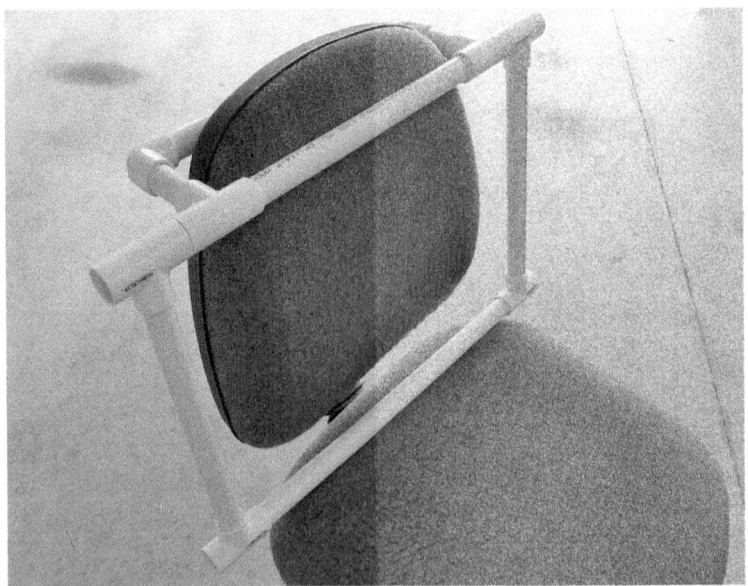

As you push the assembly down, it should fit securely on the chair back, and sit about three inches below the top. The bottom of this assembly should rest on the chair seat.

If your chair has arms, it may have to rest on the arms, rather than on the chair seat.

This Will Be the Base

The CHAIR MOUNT will be the base for a 48-inch pipe frame, on which you can hang fabric or a large photo print.

The rectangle at the rear should fit securely when you slide it over the chair back and push it down.

STEP TWO - Cut four pieces of pipe so that when they're inserted in the tees at the top and bottom of the CHAIR MOUNT, the total width from side to side is 48 inches.

Then connect those horizontal pieces with two vertical pieces so the CHAIR MOUNT looks like this:

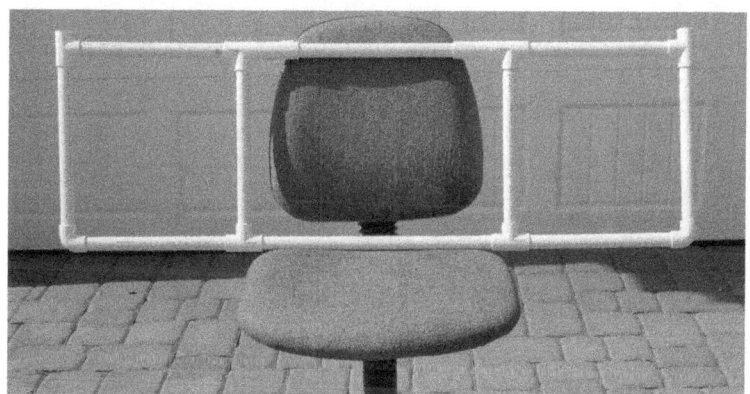

STEP THREE - Create the top of the frame with a piece of pipe that's 48 inches wide with legs about 30 inches high.

Size to Fit Your Camera Shot

You may want the frame to be a little shorter or taller, depending on the way your webcam frames the shot when you're sitting in the chair, talking on camera.

If you plan to remove the top part of the frame for storage, put some screws in tees and elbows in both the upper and lower sections.

Hammering the top part into the lower part - and then hammering again to remove it - will mess up the sections unless the screws are in place to keep them intact.

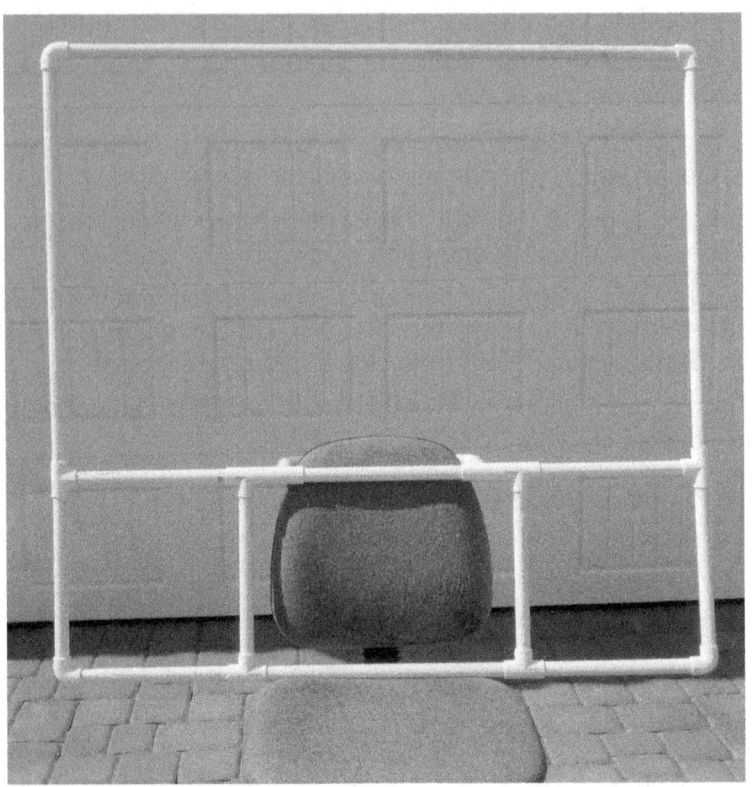

Full Chair-Mounted Frame

Here's the completed project. One of your first reactions may be:

> "Isn't that pipe in the middle of my back going to be uncomfortable?"

No.

Because when you're on camera, you should sit up straight, so your back never touches the chair.

Makes you look alert. Awake. Intelligent.

All anchors are trained to sit this way. Learn how to do it in the chapter on *News Media Interviews.*

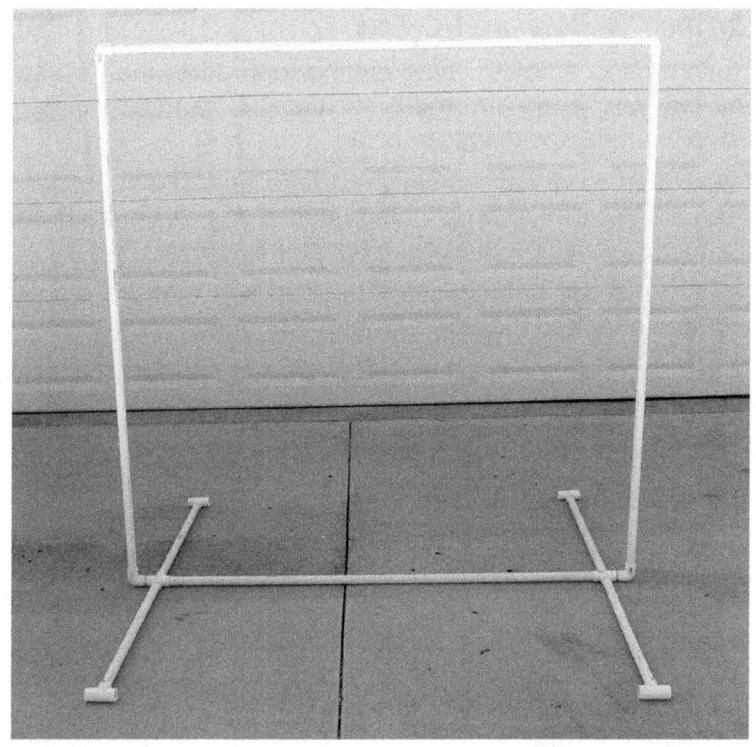

Free-Standing Frame

Here's another frame that's free-standing. It can be left in place, or dis-assembled for storage after each use.

The fabric for either frame can be a lightweight blanket of any shade or color. A twin-size blanket will give you enough coverage for a frame that's five feet square.

See more about the importance of the background in the *Lighting and Background* chapter.

Materials & Tools You'll Need

All PVC pipe and fittings for these frames is ¾ inch, Schedule 40. The pipe comes in 10-foot lengths. You can buy pipe by the foot, but it's cheaper to buy entire lengths and cut it yourself.

There's another version of PVC pipe for drains. It's thinner, and will sag. Use the heavier Schedule 40.

Cut the Pipe With a PVC Tool

I recommend a scissor-type cutting tool rather than a saw. The cut is cleaner, and more accurate. A hammer will help with assembly and disassembly.

If you plan to dis-assemble the frame and store the parts when it's not in use, You'll also need a drill, a ⅛ - inch drill bit, a screw driver, and about a dozen #8 screws.

The screws will be necessary to keep some of the elbows and tees attached through all that hammering.

At the store, they'll cut the 10-foot pipe in half for free, so it will fit in your car.

PVC Pipe & Fittings Needed (about $10)

3 pieces of pipe 10-foot- long, ¾-inch PVC pipe

10 ninety-degree elbows (much cheaper if you buy a plumber's bag of 10)

10 tees (a bag of 10)

2 four-way connectors (needed only for the free-standing frame)

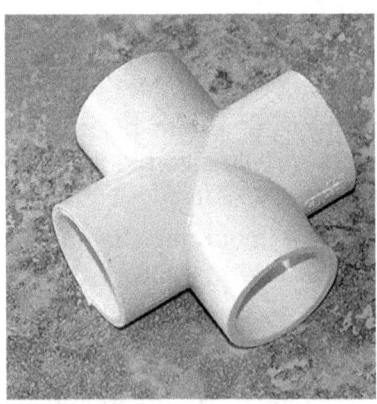

Four-Way Connectors

All stores don't stock the four-way connectors. (above) If you don't find them, you can use regular tees instead to make cross-legs that keep the frame upright.

Assembling the Frame

The module for the chair-back mount is easy because it's small. The size of the free-standing frame makes it clumsy and more difficult.

Put the parts on a level surface (the garage floor, or your driveway) stand on the pipe, and drive the elbows onto the pipes. It should lie flat.

If it's not quite square, stand on a corner or tap it with the hammer to bring it into line. The pipe and fittings are very tough. You can't hurt them.

With the free-standing frame, notice how the bottom pipe is connected to the other sides of the frame. A two-inch piece of pipe connects the four-way connector to each elbow.

With the four-sided assembly still lying flat, tap a 24-inch pipe into two of the four-way connectors.

Now It Will Stay Upright

Now you can raise the assembly and it will stay upright while you tap the remaining 24-inch pipes into the opposite sides of the four-ways.

Tees go on each end of the 24-inch pipes and are secured with screws. Their function is to help you disassemble the frame. PVC pipe, once it's tapped into a fitting, can be difficult to remove.

Hammer to Assemble or Take Apart

But it will come apart easily with a tap of your hammer on one of those tees. Or by inserting a screwdriver in one of the tees and turning it. Twisting a pipe in a fitting makes it easy to remove.

The 24-inch pipes become the base to keep the frame stable. You might be able to shorten them and maintain stability, if you don't have enough room where you're using the frame.

Any portions of the frame you don't want to disassemble when you tap a fitting should be held in place with #8 screws, ¾-inch long. Drill a ⅛-inch hole through both the fitting and the pipe to take the screws.

Don't Glue Parts Together

Don't be tempted to use PVC glue. Glued fittings won't hold if you tap them very much in assembly and disassembly.

One spot that will definitely need screws for the free-standing frame is the elbow at each end of the bottom pipe. This is where the frame will have the most stress to stay up-right with fabric attached.

Bundling the Parts for Storage

When disassembled, you can bundle the pipes together for storage. If the five-foot length won't fit your storage space, cut each of the long pipes in half and use a connector fitting to bring the bundle down to 30 inches long.

Any fabric can be draped over the top of the frame and held in place with clothespins, safety pins, or large binder clips available at office supply stores.

Weight at the Bottom of Your Fabric

You may also want to use weighted binder clips attached to the bottom of the fabric to make any wrinkles less noticea-ble. If you have enough fabric left at the bottom, you can al-so hold it down and keep it taut with books and other stuff.

A lightweight blanket works fine. I sometimes use a piece of heavier, terrycloth black fabric when I want the backdrop to be less visible.

Distance Between Backdrop & Webcam

Place the backdrop as far away from the webcam as possi-ble, still keeping the edges of the frame out of your webcam shot.

The distance helps with shadows, and will perhaps put the backdrop out of focus (see more on focus and depth of field in the *Lighting and Background* chapter).

It would be ideal to have you in sharp focus and the back-ground fuzzy. But the automatic exposure in most webcams doesn't give you a lot of control over that.

About the Author

Clarence Jones is an on-camera coach. He learned a lot about interviewing as a newspaper reporter, and then became one of the most-honored reporters in American television.

After reporting for 30 years, he wrote a book on the subject - *Winning with the News Media - A Self Defense Manual When You're the News*. The book immediately took off, and he left reporting to launch a consulting firm that specializes in on-camera training of executives in government and corporate America.

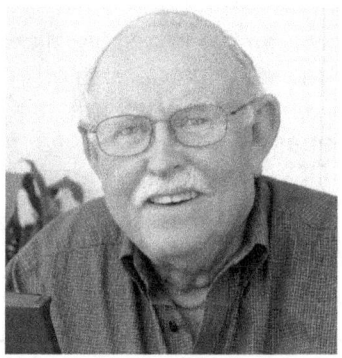

His day job Is CEO of that company. He runs Winning News Media out of a home office in Bradenton, on the west coast of Florida. He has published six other non-fiction books (listed below) and has just finished a novel (his first) in which a TV investigative reporter tries to solve the kidnap-murder of a child in Miami.

They say novelists should write about topics they know really well.

Clarence is deeply disturbed by the decline of the news media in America. The kind of reporting he did is now virtually extinct at local TV stations.

Decline of the News Media

To deal with declining profits and audiences, TV news at both the local and network levels have severely slashed both their staffs and their equipment. Webcams can save them so much money, they will soon be the norm for most local TV stations.

He wrote his first *Webcam Savvy* book to help improve the quality of those news interviews.

Job Interviews by Webcam

Webcams are also becoming standard as a screening tool for job interviews.

For job hunters, auditioning is stressful enough, without the added element of this new technology. Hopefully, his book will help level that playing field.

Starting as a Newspaper Reporter

Clarence started working for a daily newspaper when he was still in college. That career lasted 16 years (*Florida Times-Union* and *Jacksonville Journal* in Gainesville, Jacksonville, and Tallahassee. Then the *Miami Herald* in Miami and Washington, DC). He was the *Herald's* Washington correspondent when TV made him an offer he couldn't refuse.

TV Investigative Reporting

He was a TV investigative reporter for 14 years (two years at WHAS-TV in Louisville, KY, 12 years at WPLG-TV in Miami).

At WPLG, he won four Emmys and three duPont-Columbia Awards (TV's equivalent of the Pulitzer Prize). For many years, he was the only reporter for a local station who had ever won three duPont-Columbias.

Several other reporters have now matched that record.

Computer Pioneer

In December, 1968, he was the first reporter in the world to use a computer to crunch data for a series of stories analyzing Criminal Court cases for the *Miami Herald*.

Clarence has been a geek most of his life. His specialty is explaining stuff so beginners can become enthusiasts.

Photographer for Life

He had a darkroom in the family bathroom when he was in the fifth grade. In his early days as a correspondent in a distant newspaper bureaus, he shot, developed and printed the photographs for his stories.

Then he transmitted them to the home office via an ancient telephone device that took 20 minutes per photo. True Stone-Age technology.

Building His Own Computers

He bought his first desktop computer in 1984. In 2006, he built a computer from scratch for the first time.

Winning with the News Media (his first book, now in its 9th Edition) is considered by many to be the "bible" in its field.

In addition to this book, his other current books (in both print and e-book formats) are:

Winning with the News Media - *A Self-Defense Manual When You're the Story*

They're Gonna Murder You - *War Stories From My Life at the News Front*

Webcam Savvy for the Job or the News

Sailboat Projects - *Clever Ideas and How to Make Them for a Pittance*

More Sailboat Projects (a sequel), and

Filming Family History - *How to Save Great Stories for Future Generations*

He frequently publishes magazine articles on sailing, photography, and home improvement ideas. Most are how-to pieces, showing creative, inexpensive ways to do it yourself.

Contact Us

You can reach author Clarence Jones:

By e-mail:

cjones@winning-newsmedia.com

By snail mail:

Clarence Jones

6907 Vista Bella Drive

Bradenton, FL 34209

By Telephone:

941.779.0242

Help With Your Webcam

He's available to help with your webcam setup, and to teach you on-camera skills.

You can place a Skype call and talk to him on-camera. For a flat fee, he will critique your setup and make suggestions for improving it.

On-Camera Coaching

He's available to be your on-camera coach. He will role-play webcam interviews with you, helping you make your on-camera presence more effective.

He also works with clients to help them manage a crisis, or to prepare for a major presentation, news interview or news conference.

###